REGAIN YOUR BRAIN

Powerful New Scientific Discoveries that Give You Back a Youthful Mind

By Peggy Sarlin

DEDICATION:

To my parents, who continue to teach me
the value of clear thinking

And to you, because you value your brain

Regain Your Brain
Powerful New Scientific Discoveries that Give You Back a Youthful Mind

By Peggy Sarlin

Published by Online Publishing & Marketing, LLC

ISBN 978-1-5323-1689-0

Printed in the United States of America

ABOUT THE AUTHOR

Peggy Sarlin is a freelance writer with a special interest in health and wellness. She wrote the first book to investigate alternative remedies for Alzheimer's disease. Published in 2012, and revised and expanded in 2016, *Awakening from Alzheimer's: How America's Most Innovative Doctors are Reversing Alzheimer's, Dementia and Memory Loss,* has informed thousands of people about safe natural options for cognitive health. Over the past several years, Peggy has journeyed tirelessly across the U.S., interviewing the world's most renowned doctors on the forefront of the war against Alzheimer's and dementia. She shared their stories with the public in two free online video series, *Awakening from Alzheimer's: The Event* and *Regain Your Brain*. Peggy is also an accomplished singer-songwriter, who records and performs in New York.

Contents

INTRODUCTION

Your mind should be just as sharp at 95 as it is at 24. Does that statement sound realistic to you? And yet, that's what Dr. Pamela Wartian Smith, an anti-aging specialist in Michigan, told me – and she has the science to back it up.

Dr. Smith is one of more than 50 experts I interviewed in my quest to bring you the latest, most effective ways to regain your brain. I traveled the country to interview some of the most eminent doctors of our time, the heroes leading the battle against cognitive decline.

Dr. Dale Bredesen, the first person to document the reversal of Alzheimer's, shared his insights with me. So did Dr. Daniel Amen, the Founder and Medical Director of The Amen Clinics, and Dr. David Perlmutter, the renowned neurologist and best-selling author. I interviewed clinical researchers, nutritionists, and dozens of innovative physicians from a wide range of specialties. And I'm honored that several patients shared their stories with me, too.

What I learned was stunning. We're in a new world in which you don't have to lose your mind as you age. The era of helplessly succumbing to memory loss, confusion, and dementia is over. You can regain your brain, starting now.

But you need a plan. And, fortunately, that's exactly what you'll find in this book. I've taken everything I've learned from these brilliant medical minds and condensed it into a workable plan for you.

A Powerful Plan to Protect and Rejuvenate Your Brain

Are you having "senior moments," in which you forget that word on the tip of your tongue, and can't recall where you put your keys? Are you in more advanced stages of cognitive decline, getting lost in familiar places and losing the ability to work? Maybe Alzheimer's runs in your family, and you're nervous that you'll get it, too. Or perhaps you've had a concussion that's affecting your ability to function.

Whatever your situation, the information here will give your brain a new lease on life. You can take immediate action and see results. Not only will your mental clarity improve, you'll also protect yourself from devastating damage down the road.

I wish I could tell you there's a magic pill that will make all your symptoms go away, but that's not the way it works. After all, you're not changing a battery here. You're fixing your brain – the awe-inspiring miracle between your ears that's firing 18 trillion times a second. You've got 100 billion brain cells that come in 10,000 varieties, forming 100 trillion connections. There's a lot going on in your head.

Let me "warn" you of some of the side effects of regaining your brain. You'll have more energy than you've felt in decades; you'll shed unwanted weight while gaining muscle; your chronic aches and pains will melt away; you'll feel happier, calmer, and more in control; and you'll look younger and feel sexier. Can you live with that?

You'll need commitment to ensure success, but I think you'll find the motivation to keep going, because you're going to feel so good. Here's to a long life of making beautiful memories that you remember!

I'd like to give special thanks to the following people for so generously sharing their time and expertise with me.

DANIEL AMEN, M.D, is the Founder and Medical Director of the Amen Clinics, and the best-selling author of *Memory Rescue* and many other books. A distinguished fellow of the American Psychiatric Association and double board-certified psychiatrist and clinical neuroscientist, Dr. Amen has amassed the world's largest database of SPECT brain scans.

BENJAMIN ASHER, M.D., a board-certified New York City otolaryngologist, has for three decades pioneered alternative ENT (Earn, Nose and Throat) treatments. He served on the faculties of the Harvard, Washington University, and Dartmouth medical schools and on the board of the American Holistic Medical Association. A former house physician for the New York City Ballet, he was also named one of America's Top Physicians by the Consumers' Research Council of America.

DALE BREDESEN, M.D., the author of the landmark book *The End of Alzheimer's,* is a globally renowned expert on the neurodegenerative mechanisms of Alzheimer's disease. He has held faculty positions at University of California, San Francisco; UCLA; and the University of California, San Diego. Dr. Bredesen directed the Program on Aging at the Burnham Institute before coming to the Buck Institute in 1998 as its founding president and CEO. He is also the chief medical officer of MPI Cognition.

MICHAEL J. BREUS, Ph.D., is a Clinical Psychologist, Diplomate of the American Board of Sleep Medicine and Fellow of The American Academy of Sleep Medicine. He serves on the clinical advisory board of *The Dr. Oz Show*, where he regularly appears, and as a sleep expert for WebMD. Dr. Breus is the author of *The Power of When* and *The Sleep Doctor's Diet Plan*.

DONNA BROWN, M.S., is a clinical nutritionist in Connecticut. She is the principal of Nutrition Kitchen LLC, her private practice dedicated to optimizing the health, lifespan, and vitality of her clients.

RICHARD P. BROWN, M.D., Associate Clinical Professor of Psychiatry at Columbia University, is one of the world's foremost experts on the use of natural supplements. Dr. Brown is the co-author of *How to Use Herbs, Nutrients and Yoga in Mental Health*, *The Rhodiola Revolution* and *The Healing Power of the Breath*.

SHARI CAPLAN, M.D. is Founder and Medical Director of VitalityMD in Toronto, Canada. Dr. Caplan worked for over 20 years at Women's College Hospital, and is one of the few Canadian physicians board-certified in anti-aging and regenerative medicine. She is also a fellow in metabolic and nutritional medicine with the Metabolic Medical Institute.

DOMINIC D'AGOSTINO, Ph.D., is an associate professor of Aging Studies at the University of South Florida College of Behavioral and Community Sciences and its Department of Molecular Pharmacology and Physiology. A leading expert on ketones, Dr. D'Agostino researches treatments and disease prevention, using ketogenic diets and supplements.

NORMAN DOIDGE, M.D., is the best-selling author of *The Brain's Way of Healing* and *The Brain That Changes Itself*, and a leading expert on brain neuroplasticity. Dr. Doidge serves on the faculty at University of Toronto Department of Psychiatry, and the research faculty at the Columbia University Center for Psychoanalytic Training and Research.

JOHN (JAY) FABER, M.D. is a clinical and forensic psychiatrist, child psychiatrist and adult psychiatrist at Amen Clinics. He has more than two decades of experience in Child Psychiatry, Adolescent Psychiatry, and Adult Psychiatry and Pharmacological Management. He is president of BrainSource.

VINCENT FORTANASCE, M.D., the author of *The Anti-Alzheimer's Prescription*, is a Clinical Professor of Neurology at USC and Medical Director of the Fortanasce & Associates Neurology Center in Arcadia, California. He is a board-certified Neurological Rehabilitation Specialist who has treated the Dalai Lama and Pope John Paul II.

MICHAEL B. FOSSEL, M.D., Ph.D., is the author of *The Telomerase Revolution*, which was selected by *The Wall Street Journal* as one of 2015's best science books. The founder of *Rejuvenation Research*, Dr. Fossel is regarded as the world's foremost expert on clinical use of telomerase for cellular senescence in age-related diseases. He earned his M.D. and Ph.D. from Stanford University.

LEO GALLAND, M.D, a board-certified internist, is a Fellow of the American College of Nutrition and the American College of Physicians, and director of the Foundation for Integrated Medicine in New York, where he maintains a private practice. He studied at Harvard and the New York University School of Medicine. For his pioneering work in integrated medicine, Dr. Galland received the Functional Medicine Linus Pauling Award.

PATRICIA L. GERBARG, M.D., is Assistant Clinical Professor of Psychiatry at New York Medical College. A graduate of Harvard Medical College, she practices Integrative Psychiatry, combining standard and complementary treatments in her practice in Kingston, New York. With her husband, Dr. Richard P. Brown, she is the co-author of *How to Use Herbs, Nutrients and Yoga in Mental Health* and *The Rhodiola Revolution*.

DEBBIE HAMPTON writes about brain health on her website, The Best Brain Possible (www.bestbrainpossible.com). A survivor of severe brain damage, she describes the methods she used for a successful recovery.

RONALD HOFFMAN, M.D., Founder and Medical Director of the Hoffman Center in New York City, is one of America's foremost complementary medicine practitioners. Dr. Hoffman is a Certified Nutrition Specialist of the American College of Nutrition and the author of several books. He hosts a nationally syndicated radio program, *Intelligent Medicine*.

DAVID KATZ, M.D., the Founding Director (1998) of Yale University's Yale-Griffin *Prevention Research Center* and current President of the *American College of Lifestyle Medicine,* earned his M.D. from the Albert Einstein College of Medicine and a Master's in public health from Yale. A Diplomate of the American Board of Internal Medicine and a board-certified specialist in Preventive Medicine/Public Health, Dr. Katz has written 15 books. His True Health Initiative, launched in 2015, seeks to make healthful lifestyle a medical reality for people worldwide.

JOSEPH MAROON, M.D., a world-renowned neurosurgeon and Medical Director of World Wrestling Entertainment and the Pittsburgh Steelers, specializes in minimally invasive surgical treatment and injuries and diseases of the brain and spine. He has authored six books, including *Square One: A Simple Guide to a Balanced Life.* As a member of the NFL Head, Neck and Spine Committee, he co–developed the ImPACT concussion test, the only FDA–approved, global standard tool to assess concussions.

ROBERT MATHIS, M.D.. is board-certified in Integrative Holistic Medicine, Anti-aging and Regenerative Medicine, and a Certified Clinical Nutritionist. Dr. Mathis has a private practice in Santa Barbara, California.

ALAN A. MAZAREK, M.D., is a board-certified neurologist and has practiced in Rockville Centre, Long Island for nearly 30 years. He is Assistant Clinical Professor of Neurology at Mount Sinai Medical Center in Manhattan, with a strong interest in Alzheimer's Disease.

AARON P. NELSON, Ph.D., is chief of psychology and neuropsychology at Boston's Brigham and Women's Hospital and an assistant professor at Harvard Medical School. He is the author of *The Harvard Medical School Guide to Achieving Optimal Memory*.

MARY T. NEWPORT, M.D., the author of *Alzheimer's Disease: What if There was a Cure?*, helped to gain worldwide attention for the role of ketones in brain health. A neonatologist and founding medical director of two newborn intensive care units, Dr. Newport discovered the healing power of coconut oil as she searched for ways to help her husband cope with Alzheimer's.

PAUL NUSSBAUM, Ph.D., a board-certified Clinical Psychologist and Geropsychologist, specializes in Neuropsychology. He is a fellow at the National Academy of Neuropsychology and the American Academy of Clinical Psychology. An Adjunct Professor of Neurological Surgery at the University of Pittsburgh School of Medicine, Dr. Nussbaum is Founder and President of Brain Health Center, Inc.

STEVEN Y. PARK, M.D., is board-certified in Sleep Medicine and Otolaryngology. An Assistant Professor of Otolaryngology at Albert Einstein College of Medicine, Dr. Park practices integrative medicine and surgery in New York. He is the author of *Sleep, Interrupted.*

DAVID PERLMUTTER, M.D., is a board-certified neurologist and a Fellow of the American College of Nutrition. His best-selling books, *Grain Brain* and *Brain Maker*, have been translated into 27 languages and helped to educate millions of people about brain health. Dr. Perlmutter received the Linus Pauling Award for his innovative approaches to neurological disorders. He lives in Naples, Florida.

FRED PESCATORE, M.D., is the Medical Director of Medicine 369 in New York, where he practices integrative medicine. Dr. Pescatore was the Associate Medical Director of The Atkins Center for Complementary Medicine and currently publishes the *Logical Health Alternatives* newsletter.

DALE PETERSON, M.D., is a past president of the Oklahoma Academy of Family Physicians. An expert on iatrogenic illness (sickness caused by medical treatment), Dr. Peterson was Chief of Staff at Edmond Hospital in Edmond, Oklahoma. He founded Wellness Clubs of America to give people access to credible information on supporting their health.

ANGELA POFF, PH.D., is a postdoctoral research fellow in the Department of Molecular Pharmacology and Physiology at the University of South Florida. She specializes in medical applications of ketosis for cancer and other illnesses.

MARY KAY ROSS, M.D., is the founder and owner of the Institute for Personalized Medicine in Savannah, Georgia. A Fellow of the American College of Emergency Physicians, Dr. Ross is affiliated with the Institute for Functional Medicine and trained with Dr. Dale Bredesen in his protocol for reversing Alzheimer's.

PAMELA WARTIAN SMITH, M.D., is the owner and director of The Center for Personalized Medicine in Michigan. She is the author of *What You Must Know About Memory Loss & How You Can Stop It* and many other books. Dr. Smith is a Diplomate of the American Academy of Anti-Aging Physicians and founder of the Fellowship in Anti-Aging, Regenerative, and Functional Medicine.

JACOB TEITELBAUM, M.D., is a board-certified internist and nationally known expert on chronic illnesses. The author of numerous books, including *Real Cause, Real Cure* and *From Fatigued to Fantastic!,* Dr. Teitelbaum is a Founding Diplomate of the American Board of Holistic Medicine and Director of the Practitioners Alliance Network (PAN).

ALLAN WARSHOWSKY, M.D., is. a board-certified OB-GYN and a founding Diplomat and Director Emeritus of the American Board of Integrative Holistic Medicine. A member of the American Holistic Association and the American Board of Obstetrics and Gynecology, Dr. Warshowsky has a private practice in Rye, New York.

CHAPTER ONE

UPGRADE YOUR SLEEP

PART ONE

WHY SLEEP?

"Do you know what's the most common cause of memory loss?" Dr. Alan Mazarek challenged me over the phone. As I racked my brain, Dr. Mazarek, a New York neurologist, supplied the answer: "*Lack of sleep*!"

If you haven't been sleeping well, join the club. An estimated 70 million Americans have sleep problems, according to the National Center on Sleep Disorders, and they're not just getting grouchier. They're also getting fatter, sicker, and dramatically more at risk of developing Alzheimer's and other forms of dementia.

Lack of Sleep like "Being Hit on the Head"

A *Daily Mail* headline tells the tale: "*A lack of sleep 'damages the brain in a similar way to being hit on the head'.*" 15 healthy young men underwent sleep studies at Sweden's Uppsala University. After just one sleepless night, they exhibited elevated levels of biochemical markers for brain damage like those caused by a blow to the head.

And if that research isn't scary enough, these sleep studies could give you nightmares:

50 percent Higher Risk of Mental Decline From Poor Sleep

- For every percentage point you lose of Rapid Eye Movement (REM) sleep, your risk of dementia increases a terrifying nine percent!

- Heavy snorers and people with sleep apnea show signs of Alzheimer's or mild cognitive impairment (MCI) a stunning **10 years earlier** than better sleepers.

- Poor quality sleep increases the risk of damaged mental capacity as much as 50 percent, **equivalent to a five year increase in age**.

Sleep Is Like Miracle-Gro For Your Brain

"Without good sleep, you age sickly and quickly," Dr. Vincent Fortanasce, the author of *The Anti-Alzheimer's Prescription,* told me. "Sleep is like Miracle-Gro for your brain." Though it may look like passive suspension, sleep is an extremely active period, in which the brain recharges.

I was curious to learn how lack of sleep affects the most famously sleep-deprived profession of all: new doctors. What I found in the article, "The Secret Horrors of Sleep-Deprived Doctors" shocked me. See for yourself…

"I was so sleep deprived that I'd fall asleep while writing patient notes and write my dreams into the notes."

"I have made numerous medication errors from being over tired. I also recently misread an EKG because I was so tired I literally couldn't see straight…She [the patient] died."

"I thought I could keep going at that pace and nothing terrible would happen until I woke up in the ICU and a doctor told me I had tried to kill myself."

All Sleep Cycles Are Not The Same

There's no escaping it: we need sleep. The best present you could give your brain tonight is eight hours of solid sleep, during which you cycle through four distinct stages.

REM (Rapid Eye Movement) sleep is your dream time. Before you get there, your brain will progress through three stages of NREM (non-REM) sleep, sinking deeper until you reach the ultimate "slow-wave" stage of N3 sleep.

But people with sleep disorders have a terrible problem: *they never get into the deeper sleep and REM stages.* Consequently, their health suffers, because each stage of sleep has its own healing powers.

Dr. Michael Breus, a prominent sleep expert in California, told me, "All sleep cycles are not the same. In the first part of the night, that's when we get more Stage 3 and 4 sleep, which is 'deep sleep' that repairs the body. In the last third of the night, we get more REM sleep, when all the mental restoration occurs."

"So if you wake up early or cut off one of the cycles, which one did you cut off? Did you cut off the deep sleep one, so that you don't feel good physically, or did you cut off the REM sleep, so you're having cognition issues?"

"When somebody comes to me and says, 'Dr Breus, I can't find my keys. I walk into a room and forget why I'm there,' *that's REM sleep deprivation*. That's not necessarily that you've got a memory or cognition issue."

Four Reasons You Need Four-Stage Sleep Tonight

Here are four huge brain benefits from a successful night of sleep:

1. Memories are consolidated during sleep.

"During REM sleep, information moves from your short-term memory to your long-term memory. That's when information gets placed into an organizational structure in your brain, so that you can retrieve it, in order to make good decisions," Dr. Breus said.

2. Vital anti-aging hormones are secreted during sleep.

"Sleep is the rhythm of the hormonal symphony," Dr. Vincent Fortanasce told me. "During deep sleep, your **serotonin and dopamine** levels increase. Those are the 'happiness hormones' that regulate your executive and calming functions."

"Also during N3 sleep, **your human growth hormone increases, which is the main hormone to keep you young**. Imagine that your body is an electric car. Sleep is when you recharge your hormones and neurotransmitters."

3. Toxins get cleared away from your brain cells during sleep.

Sleep is waste removal time for your brain. During deep sleep, your brain cells shrink, allowing space for fluids to enter and wash away toxic waste.

"The brain only has limited energy at its disposal and it appears that it must choose between two different functional states - awake and aware or asleep and cleaning up," said researcher Dr. Maiken Nedergaard, who conducted a University of Rochester study on brain cell shrinkage during sleep.

"You can think of it like having a house party. You can either entertain the guests or clean up the house, but you can't really do both at the same time. The housekeeping function of sleep may be vital to warding off Alzheimer's, which is characterized by a buildup of toxic protein in the brain."

4. Sleep invigorates your cellular energy.

Sleep energizes your mitochondria, the energy furnaces burning in every cell in your body. An important 2015 study in Denmark of identical twins found that if they often under-slept, the mitochondrial numbers in their blood cells plummeted.

"When the twins slept for 90 minutes less than they should – for a prolonged period – their cell function seemed to be reduced to a level equivalent to that of someone ten years older," said the study's co-author.

PART TWO

STOP BAD HABITS THAT CAUSE BAD SLEEP

Do you fall asleep, but can't stay asleep? Are you up every night till 2 A.M.? Do you sleep fitfully for eight hours, and then wake up exhausted? What's stopping you from getting the sleep you need?

Why Aren't You Getting Good Sleep?

It turns out there's an art and science to getting a good night's sleep, but many of its requirements aren't obvious. You could easily do a dozen things today that will steal your sleep tonight, without realizing it.

BAD HABIT #1: EATING THE WRONG THINGS AT THE WRONG TIME

You think a lot about how diet affects your weight. But do you ever consider how your food choices influence your sleep? In fact, what you eat – and when you eat it – can make a huge difference in the quality of your nightly rest.

How many of these bad bedtime habits do you have?

SUGAR: "Sugar is a shock to your system," says Dr. Steven Y. Park, a New York sleep surgeon and author of *Sleep, Interrupted*. "If you have a large amount of sugar, your body will pump out lots of insulin, which will cause a bad night's sleep."

And Dr. Park warns that once you're sleep-deprived, you're more likely to choose junk food the next day, continuing the vicious cycle.

BOTTOM LINE: For sweet dreams, ditch the sweets.

AFTERNOON CAFFEINE: According to Michigan researchers, **drinking coffee even six hours before bedtime reduced nightly sleep by more than one hour**.

And if you're sensitive to caffeine, its buzz may last up to eleven or twelve hours. That's why I've learned to enjoy my one precious cup of java before noon.

REMINDER: Tea, cola, and chocolate contain caffeine, too.

AN ALCOHOLIC NIGHTCAP: A major five-year study of alcohol and sleep at the University of Missouri School of Medicine prompted its co-author, Dr. Pradeep Sahota, to report:

"It's clear that alcohol should not be used as a sleep aid. Alcohol disrupts sleep and the quality of sleep is diminished. Additionally, alcohol is a diuretic, which increases your need to go the bathroom and causes you to wake up earlier in the morning."

BIG MEALS BEFORE BED: When you eat a lot before bedtime, your body has to work hard to digest it – too hard to relax into deep sleep. "A lot of people don't eat much for breakfast or lunch, and then they have this really big dinner. It's like a rock in their stomach, and it takes the body a lot to metabolize through that," Dr. Breus told me.

To promote sleep, try eating a lunch-sized dinner and a dinner-sized lunch. For an even bigger health boost, aim for at least a 12-hour window between dinner and breakfast. For instance, if you finish eating dinner at 8 P.M., don't eat again till at least 8 A.M. Go for even longer, if you can. These fasting stretches promote deeper sleep and better health.

BAD HABIT#2: STIMULATING THOSE NIGHTTIME BATHROOM TRIPS

You'll sleep better if you don't keep waking up to go to the bathroom. Here are six simple tips to combat this annoying problem.

1. **Watch your fluids before bedtime**: Cut out all drinks an hour or two before bed.

2. **Limit foods that irritate your bladder**: Potential irritants include tomato products; coffee and tea; chocolate; citrus fruits; adult beverages; carbonated drinks; spicy foods; sweeteners; processed foods; raw onions; and cranberries. Keep a food diary to determine which foods affect you most.

3. **Prop up your feet on a pillow**: Encourage fluid to drain from your legs by propping them on a pillow during the evening. Empty your bladder before bedtime and enjoy a longer stretch of sleep. (This tip comes Dr. Jacob Teitelbaum, an alternative medicine expert.)

4. **Attend to any underlying infections**: Are you harboring a simmering yeast or urinary tract infection? They could be irritating your bladder, so make sure to clear them up.

5. **Consider trying an Icelandic plant extract**: Dr. Teitelbaum told me about SagaPro, which is extracted from the Icelandic plant *angelica archangelica*, and supports bladder strength. SagaPro is available online, where I found lots of positive user reviews.

6. **Consider trying Saw Palmetto**: This herb enjoys a big reputation for helping prostate problems, although clinical trials are mixed about its results. Dr. Teitelbaum recommends 160 mg twice a day.

† **NOTE:** Saw palmetto is generally considered safe, but should not be used during pregnancy or breastfeeding. Stop usage two weeks before surgery, since it may slow blood clotting.

BAD HABIT #3: NOT GETTING ENOUGH SUNLIGHT

Your body is designed to wake up in the morning with the sun and to sleep when it gets dark. If you miss out on sunlight, particularly morning sunlight, you can confuse your inner clock.

Dr. Park told me about a sick, overweight patient with bad sleep habits. "I advised her not to drink alcohol late and to exercise outside in the morning. Well, she just wrote me that she lost 30 pounds and ran the New York City marathon!"

Get up, get out, and get moving in the morning sun to deepen your sleep at night.

BAD HABIT #4: IGNORING SNORING

Do you have **sleep apnea**? Here are some signs: 1) loud, persistent snoring 2) pauses in breathing that cause you to wake up gasping 3) frequent fatigue during the day.

Sleep Apnea Can Be Fatal

Dr. Breus told me, "Sleep apnea is actually a blockage of the throat, with no oxygen going in. When that occurs, your heart slows down to conserve the oxygen in the system."

"Then your brain says, 'Oh, my gosh, there's no air!' It makes the heart beat faster to wake you up. So your heart rate is slowing down, speeding up."

"It puts an extra load on the heart, and that can cause something called 'refractory hypertension,' which is high blood pressure that doesn't work for pills. The only way to treat those patients is to treat their sleep apnea."

Alzheimer's Patients Are Five Times More Likely to Have Sleep Apnea

The connection between sleep apnea and Alzheimer's is well documented. In 2016, a group of scientists published a review of the medical literature on this topic, and reached a frightening conclusion:

"…patients with AD [Alzheimer's Disease] have a five times higher chance of presenting with OSA [Obstructive Sleep Apnea] than cognitively non-impaired individuals of similar age."

Now that's scary. Alzheimer's patients are *five times* more likely to have sleep apnea! That's a wake-up call to treat it, with your doctor's help.

The Gold Standard Sleep Apnea Treatment

The gold standard for treating sleep apnea is the CPAP (Continuous Positive Airway Pressure), which requires a face or nasal mask, connected to a pump.

"CPAP is a little air compressor, like a hair dryer. It shoots a thin stream of air through a tube with a little mask that sits on your nose. When it hits that area, it just ever so slightly opens it up. It doesn't hurt. It doesn't have any side effects. It's not the sexiest thing in the world, but it works," Dr. Breus told me.

Provent, a New Disposable Alternative for Treating Apnea

Dr. Benjamin Asher, a leading holistic ear, nose and throat specialist in New York, told me about Provent, a disposable alternative to the CPAP that requires no mask or machine. It works by attaching to your nostrils, and creating pressure to keep the airway open when you exhale. Learn more at www.proventtherapy.com.

Easy Options for Clearing Nasal Congestion

"Your quality of sleep goes downhill when you have nasal congestion. So whatever is causing it, deal with it immediately," Dr. Park advises. Here are some simple devices that may increase airflow through your nose, for as little as 37 cents a night.

Breathe Right Nasal Strips: "If you take 100 people and give them Breathe Rights Strips, ten of them will get amazing sleep," he said. "Try the Breathe Right Strips and **Nasal Saline Irrigation** (neti pot). Do them both before bed."

NoZoVent and Sinus Cones: These nasal dilators are designed to comfortably widen the nostril and increase airflow. "Many options are available online of strips that pull apart the nostrils from the outside or the inside," notes Dr. Park. "These are two good ones." You can find NoZoVent at **NoSnoreZone.com**

BAD HABIT #5: SLEEPING IN THE WRONG POSITION

Most doctors don't appreciate the importance of a proper sleep position, says Dr. Park. He recently saw a middle-aged patient with serious memory problems and exhaustion. It turned out that two months earlier, her dermatologist had told her to sleep on her back, instead of stomach, to avoid wrinkles. "I told her the whole incident was brought on by artificially forcing herself to sleep in an unnatural position," Dr. Park told me.

He added that chiropractors sometimes tell people to avoid sleeping on their side or stomach. But many people can't sleep successfully on their back.

Dr. Park advises people to regain their sleep position after surgery as soon as possible. "If you have surgery, you're given a narcotic. That depresses your respiratory drive, so you're breathing less." Getting back to your natural sleep position will help to restore proper breathing.

BAD HABIT #6: SCREEN GAZING BEFORE BED

It's one A.M. and you're still on Facebook. And it's not because you're hooked on photos of your cousin's dog. Your computer screen is emitting blue light that may be disrupting your sleep. And so is your tablet. And cell phone. And Kindle. And TV.

"Any light lowers melatonin levels," Dr. Park told me. "The new screens have extra blue light, and we know that blue light suppresses melatonin levels and, therefore, sleep."

Melatonin is a master hormone that commands your sleep and wake cycles. In the evening, levels rise to promote sleep. In the morning, levels drop, prodding you awake.

Bedtime Screens Lower Melatonin by 55 Percent

A 2015 study published in PNAS (Proceedings of the National Academy of Sciences) had bad news for bedtime E-readers. Not only did iPad users **produce 55 percent less melatonin when reading at night**, they had less REM sleep and took "hours longer" to feel alert the next morning.

Most experts I talked to urge the avoidance of backlit devices for two hours before bedtime. But if giving up your electronic toys seems impossible, you can at least make some improvements in your situation.

Clever Ways to Limit Dangerous Blue Light

The problems that technology created, new technology can help to solve. A host of clever new products has emerged to shield your eyes from blue light waves.

f.lux: This software automatically filters out blue light in the evening from your screen. You can download f.lux software for a variety of computers, iPhones and iPads. Check out justgetflux.com.

Ocushield.com products are anti-blue light protectors that you physically attach to your screen. Or you can get blue-light blocking glasses to wear in the evening at **LowBlueLights.com.**

GE Align Bulbs aim to "avoid disrupting the body's natural circadian rhythms" with one bulb for daylight and another for evening. **Hue bulbs** come with an app that lets you adjust your bulbs' color spectrum.

Lights Out In Your Bedroom

Now that you've blocked your blue light problem, take a fresh look around your bedroom. Is your sleep environment as pitch-black as you can make it?

"See what you can do to cover up lights. I found that it works to block LED lights with black electric tape. And if you're in a hotel room with a bright alarm clock, cover it with a towel," Dr. Park advised.

Dr. Allan B. Warshowsky, an integrative physician in Rye, New York, told me, "**Cover your electrical appliances**. This is very important, because they will interrupt sleep. Even the electromagnetic waves that come from cable boxes could disrupt sleep."

PART THREE

THE SHOCKING FACTS ABOUT SLEEPING PILLS

54-year-old Kerry Kennedy looked chagrined as she stood before the judge, facing charges of driving while impaired. The daughter of Robert Kennedy had slammed into a tractor-trailer after driving erratically on a New York highway.

But she was soon grinning when a jury acquitted her, based on blood tests showing she had taken Ambien, a prescription sleeping medication.

At least 8.6 million Americans take prescribed sleeping pills, so Kennedy isn't the only sedative user endangering people on the road.

Car Crash Risk Doubles for Sleeping Pill Users

A recent study in the American Journal of Public Health exposed the frightening dangers of Ambien, Restoril, Oleptrol and Desyril, the most commonly prescribed sleep aids.

Users of these pills were **twice** as likely to be involved in car crashes, especially in the morning when the sedative effect lingered in the bloodstream. Their risk of accidents equaled that of drunk drivers.

"This finding is shockingly not shocking. Sleeping pills are a huge problem," according to Dr. Christopher Winter, a spokesman for the American Academy of Sleep Medicine. "This study screams that many doctors do not know how to treat sleep patients," he said. "You have to develop a plan to deal with their sleep, not merely sedate them."

Warning: Ambien Sends More Seniors to the ER Than Any Other Drug

Older patients who take sleeping pills are more at risk of falls and fractures, and resulting hospitalization, according to researchers at the Centers for Disease Control and Johns Hopkins.

In fact, **Ambien – just by itself – accounted for one out of five emergency room visits among those older than 65**. Now that's a stunning statistic! *In fact, Ambien is the medication most responsible for sending seniors to the emergency room.*

Dr. Lee Hampton, lead author of the C.D.C. study, commented, "Often, in medicine, the easiest thing doctors can do is write a prescription. Things that take longer and require more conversation are used less."

I asked Dr. Breus about the risks of Ambien and other prescription sleeping drugs. "When you look at the data very closely, it turns out that a lot of people mix alcohol with the sleep aid," he replied. "That's when the problems occur."

The Biggest Reason People Don't Sleep: Anxiety or Depression

Dr. Breus explained to me that sleeping pills are often prescribed for psychological problems, not physical ones. "There's a mental aspect to sleep. 75 percent of the reason why people either don't fall asleep or stay asleep is either anxiety or depression."

"So the doctor gives them a pill, which makes them fall asleep. And the resulting dependence on the sleeping pill is psychological, not physical."

Common Medications That Sabotage Sleep

When I read the horrifying statistic about Ambien accounting for 20 percent of emergency room visits by seniors, I had an unsettling thought. How many of those patients were taking Ambien to counteract the insomnia brought on by their other medications?

It's an unhappy fact that many common prescription medications can induce insomnia. And all too often, both doctors and patients underestimate the havoc on sleep created by these popular pharmaceutical drugs.

Are You Taking Any of These Medications?

Dr. Armon B. Neel, Jr., PharmD, CGP, writing for AARP, described ten types of medications that can cause sleep problems.

1. Alpha-blockers
Prescribed for high blood pressure, enlarged prostate, and Reynaud's disease. Some brand names: Uroxatral, Cardura, Minipress, Rapaflo, Hytrin and Flomax.

2. Beta-blockers

Used to treat high blood pressure and arrhythmias (irregular heartbeat). Some brand names: Tenormin, Coreg, Lopressor, Toprol, Inderal, Betapace, and Timoptic.

3. Corticosteroids

Prescribed for rheumatoid arthritis, lupus, gout, allergic reactions, and inflammation of blood vessels and muscles. Some brand names: Medrol, Deltasone and Sterapred.

4. SSRI antidepressants

Prescribed for depression. Some brand names: Prozac, Sarafem, Celexa, Lexapro, Paxil, Pexeva, Zoloft.

5. ACE inhibitors

Prescribed for high blood pressure, congestive heart failure and other conditions. Some brand names: Lotensin, Capoten, Vasotec, Monopril, Prinivil, Zestrel, Univasc, Aceon, Accupril, Altace, Mavik.

6. ARBs (Angiotensin II-receptor blockers)

Used for coronary artery disease, heart failure, type 2 diabetes and kidney disease. Some brand names: Atacand, Avapro, Cozaar, Micardis, Diovan.

7. Cholinesterase inhibitors

Used for memory loss in patients with Alzheimer's and dementia. Some brand names: Aricept, Razadyne, and Exelon.

IRONY ALERT: I must pause here to point out the horrible irony. If you take any of these cholinesterase inhibitors for Alzheimer's or dementia, they could sabotage your sleep – and, therefore, **increase** your memory problems. In other words, they could worsen the very symptoms that you're taking them for.

8. Second-generation (non-sedating) H1 antagonists

Prescribed as antihistamines to counter the symptoms of allergic reactions. Some brand names: Astelin, Zyrtec, Claritin, Clarinex, Allegra, Xyzal.

9. Glucosamine and chondroitin

Dietary supplements used to treat joint pain and inflammation. The Federal Drug Administration classifies these substances as foods, not drugs.

Dr. Neel recommends that you take glucosamine in the morning, because it has a longer half-life in the body than chondroitin. Hopefully, a morning dose will not promote insomnia.

10. Statins

Prescribed for high cholesterol. Some brand names: Lipitor, Mevacor, Vytorin, Zocor

Statins have been linked in a number of studies with memory loss. Perhaps their disruption of sleep may be a contributing cause.

Breaking the Vicious Cycle of Medications that Disrupt Sleep

Dr. Neel suggests that if you take any of these drugs and suffer from sleeplessness, consult your doctor and pharmacist. They may be able to swap the medication, adjust the dosage, or suggest different schedules for taking them.

Best of all, your health provider may recommend a non-prescription therapy, such as a change of diet, increased exercise, or a natural supplement.

PART FOUR

SAFE NATURAL AIDS FOR BLISSFUL SLEEP

Occasionally you may want to take a safe, natural sleep supplement. I plunged into the research and also asked several of the most respected integrative doctors to share their suggestions.

MELATONIN: MASTER HORMONE OF YOUR INTERNAL CLOCK

Melatonin often pops up first in recommendations for sleep supplements, because of its starring role in regulating the sleep and wake cycle. As nighttime approaches, your melatonin level rises, signaling your brain: "Hey, go to sleep."

Unfortunately, when you hit your senior years, melatonin levels decline, making supplements a tempting option.

Safety Advice About Taking Melatonin

But melatonin supplements come with risks. "Melatonin is a hormone. You wouldn't go down to your local health food store and buy testosterone or estrogen. Those are pretty well-controlled substances. But melatonin is not well-controlled," Dr. Breus told me.

He explained that the quality of commercial melatonin varies widely, and that 95 percent of the melatonin supplements are sold in overdose formats.

"Normal adult dosage is going to be between a half and one milligram – that's it. But most melatonin supplements are sold in 3, 5, or 10 milligrams," Dr. Breus said.

If you want to try melatonin, consider following the advice of Ray Sahelian, M.D., an expert on supplements. In his book *Mind Boosters*, Dr. Sahelian wrote that he's been taking 0.3 to 1 milligram of melatonin once or twice a week for years. He advises keeping the dose that low and not using it more than twice a week.

WARNING: **Check with your doctor to make sure that melatonin will not negatively interact with your medications.** Melatonin is not advised if you take blood thinners, immunosuppressants, or diabetes medications, among others.

MAKE YOURSELF A DELICIOUS CUP OF BANANA TEA

Healthy magnesium levels can really help you sleep. In the chapter on stress, I discuss several ways to take magnesium, which can be tricky.

Here's a different approach that I learned from Dr. Breus. As bedtime approaches, brew yourself a cup of banana tea. "Bananas are loaded with magnesium," he explained. "And the peel of the banana has three times the magnesium as the fruit. Wash the banana and cut off the tips. Cut the banana in half, leaving the peel. Put it in boiling water for four to five minutes till it turns brown. It's very calming."

VALERIAN: THE PLANT ROOTS THAT SOOTHE AND CALM

Valerian is an ancient sedative, used for both anxiety and insomnia. Its roots are often combined with other herbs in commercial sleeping aids. Studies indicate that valerian gains effectiveness with continuous nightly use, instead of as an occasional sleep aid. The FDA classifies valerian as GRAS (generally recognized as safe).

DOSE: Dr. Jacob Teitelbaum recommends a dose of 200 to 500 milligrams. Higher doses of 450 to 900 milligrams can make you groggy the next day. He notes that ten percent of people experience valerian as a stimulant. In that case, only take it for daytime anxiety.

GLYCINE: THE TINY AMINO ACID THAT NORMALIZES SLEEP ARCHITECTURE

Glycine is the tiniest amino acid, but it plays a big role in building protein and transmitting chemical messages in the brain. Now glycine is gaining recognition for its usefulness in promoting sleep. According to Tamara Eriksen, N.D., "At moderate doses, glycine supplementation can help normalize sleep architecture to restore the myriad benefits of restful, restorative sleep."

DOSE: 3 grams daily, at bedtime

Dr. Ronald Hoffman, an integrative physician in New York, told me about **Glysom**, which processes glycine into a lemon-flavored powder. According to Dr. Hoffman, Glysom is safe for nightly consumption.

IMPORTANT SAFETY WARNINGS:

If you've been taking prescription sleeping pills for more than a month, work with your doctor to taper them off, rather than going cold turkey.

Talk to your physician about possible interactions with other medications. Be aware that many supplements are not recommended for use if you're pregnant or nursing. Check the cautionary notes on the labels.

PART FIVE

WHAT YOU CAN DO;
WHAT YOUR DOCTOR CAN DO

"Sleep that knits up the ravell'd sleeve of care"
— William Shakespeare

WHAT YOU CAN DO

1. **Make getting sleep a top priority.** Aim for at least seven hours, and set a consistent schedule of when you wake up and go to bed.

2. **Soak up the sun, especially in the morning**. Sunlight establishes the rhythm of your sleep/wake cycle. Walk in the morning to sleep better at night.

3. **Change your bedroom into a sleep-friendly environment.** Keep the room dark and cool. Cover up the lights from your clock, phone, power-strip, television, etc.

4. **Avoid stimulants before bed**. Steer clear of vigorous exercise, caffeine, alcohol, nicotine, heavy food, sugar, and watching the news.

5. **Create a relaxing bedtime ritual**. Take a hot bath, do some gentle stretches, meditate, breathe, read. Try making a cup of banana tea.

6. **Calm your mind by counting backwards from 300 by threes.** If your mind is agitated, this simple trick calms you down. According to Dr. Breus, "it's mathematically so complicated that you can't think of anything else, and it's so doggone boring, you're out like a light."

7. Deal with underlying medical issues that may contribute to sleeplessness.

8. Get treated for sleep apnea, if appropriate. Sleep apnea is dangerous: you stop breathing and your throat actually collapses. You need to take care of it right away, before it creates long-term damage to your health.

WHAT YOUR DOCTOR CAN DO

1. Review your medications to see if they could cause insomnia. Advise about sleep supplements you are considering taking.

2. Treat underlying conditions that may hurt sleep. Medical sleep-busters include:

1. Chronic Pain

2. Sleep apnea

3. Obesity

4. Adrenal Stress

5. Testosterone deficiency

6. Menopausal hormones

7. Depression

8. Sinus problems, congestion, allergies

9. Hypoglycemia

3. Evaluate you for sleep apnea and recommend appropriate treatment. If necessary, your doctor can refer you to a sleep clinic.

NOTES:

Part One:

"National Institute of Health Sleep Disorders Research Plan," National Center on Sleep Disorders Research, National Institutes of Health, Nov. 2011, https://www.nhlbi.nih.gov/files/docs/resources/sleep/201101011NationalSleepDisordersResearchPlanDHHSPublication11-7820.pdf.

"A lack of sleep 'damages the brain in a similar way to being hit on the head'," *Daily Mail*, Dec. 31, 2013, last consulted Dec, 2017.

J. Cedernaes, ME Osler, et al, "Acute Sleep Loss Induces Tissue-Specific Epigenetic and Transcriptional Alterations to Circadian Clock Genes in Men," *Journal of Clinical Endochrinology and Metabolism*, Sept. 2015.

Ricardo S. Osorio, Tyler Gumb, et al, "Sleep-disordered breathing advances cognitive decline in the elderly," *Neurology*, April 15, 2015.

"Heavy snoring, sleep apnea may signal earlier memory and thinking decline," *Science Daily*, Apr. 15, 2015.

Emma Innes, "How a bad night's sleep could age your brain by five years: poor quality slumber causes loss of memory and concentration," *Daily Mail*, Apr. 1, 2014.

Terri Blackwell, MA, Kristine Yaffe, MD, et al, "Associations of Objectively and Subjectively Measured Sleep Quality with Subsequent Cognitive Decline in Older Community-Dwelling Men: The MrOS Sleep Study," *Sleep*, Vol. 37, No. 4, Apr. 1, 2014.

A M Williamson, Anne-Marie Feyer, "Moderate sleep deprivation produces impairments in cognitive and motor performance equivalent to legally prescribed levels of alcohol intoxication," *Occupational and Environmental Medicine*, Vol. 57, No. 10, Oct. 2000.

"Less REM sleep tied to greater risk of dementia," *Science Daily*, Aug. 23, 2017.

Matthew P. Pase, PhD, Jayandra J. Himali, et al, "Sleep architecture and the risk of incident dementia in the community," *Neurology*, Aug. 2017.

Dr. Vincent Fortanasce, *The Anti-Alzheimer's Prescription*, (Avery, August 4, 2009).

Pamela Wible, MD, "The Secret Horrors of Sleep-Deprived Doctors," *KevinMD*, Mar. 12, 2017, https://www.kevinmd.com/blog/2017/03/secret-horrors-sleep-deprived-doctors.html.

Karen Debas, Julie Carrier, et al. "Off-line consolidation of motor sequence learning results in greater integration within a cortico-striatal functional network," *NeuroImage*, Vo. 99, Oct. 1, 2014.

Pam Harrison, "Sleep on it: sleep consolidates memory of new motor task," *Medscape Medical News*, Sept. 8, 2014.

"To Sleep, Perchance to Clean," University of Rochester Medical Center, Oct. 17, 2013.

L. Xie, H. Kang, et al, "Sleep drives metabolite clearance from the adult brain," *Science*, Science, Oct. 18, 2013.

Arianna Huffington, "If You Value Your Brain, Get More Sleep," *The Sleep Revolution: Transforming Your Life, One Night at a Time,* (Harmony, Apr. 5, 2016), as excerpted in "Are Your Sleep Habits Messing with Your Mental Health?" at *Nutritious Life.*

Bo Christensen, "How poor sleep affects your body," *ScienceNordic*, Nov. 6, 2015.

Joanna E. Wrede, MD, Jonas Mengel-From, Ph.D., Msc, et al, "Mitochondrial DNA Copy Number in Discordant Monozygotic Twins," *Sleep*, Vol. 38, No. 10, Oct. 1, 2015.

Part Two:

Dr. Steven Y. Park, *Sleep, Interrupted: A Physician Reveals the #1 Reason Why So Many of Us are Sick and Tired* (Jodev Press, Fe, 9, 2012).

T. Drake, Roehrs, et al, "Caffeine effects on sleep taken 0, 3, or 6 hours before going to bed," *Journal of Clinical Sleep Medicine*, Nov. 15, 2013.

Catherine Paddock, Ph.D., "Alcohol disrupts body's sleep regulator," *Medical News Today*, Dec. 11, 2014.

Ryan Wallace, "11 foods to avoid if you have OAB," *HealthLine*, Oct. 3, 2016, https://www.healthline.com/health/11-foods-to-avoid-if-you-have-oab.

Dr. Jacob Teitelbaum and Bill Gottleib, *Real Cause, Real Cure: the 9 root causes of the most common health problems*, (Rodale Press, Aug. 7, 2012).

Farnoosh Emamian, Habibolah Khazaie, et al, "The Association between obstructive sleep apnea and Alzheimer's disease: a meta-analysis perspective," *Frontiers in Aging Neuroscience*, Apr. 12, 2016.

B. Wood, MS Rea, et al, "Light level and duration of exposure determine the impact of self-luminous tablets on melatonin suppression," *Applied Ergonomics*, Mar. 2013.

Anne-Marie Changa, Daniel Aeschbacha, et al, "Evening use of light-emitting eReaders negatively affects sleep, circadian timing, and next-morning alertness," *Proceedings of the National Academy of Sciences*, vol. 112, no. 4, Jan. 27, 2015.

Part Three:

Maggie Fox, "Sleeping pill use raises car crash risk, study finds," *NBC News*, Jun. 11, 2015.

Stephen Reinberg, "Car crash risk doubles for users of sleeping pills, study finds," *Health Day*, Jun. 11, 2015.

Ryan N. Hansen, Denise M. Boudreau, et al, "Sedative Hypnotic Medication Use and the Risk of Motor Vehicle Crash," *American Journal of Public Health*, Apr. 15, 2015.

Paula Span, "More on sleeping pills and older adults," *New York Times*, Jul. 30, 2014.

Lee M. Hampton, M.D., Matthew Daudresse, et al, "Emergency Department Visits by Adults for Psychiatric Medication Adverse Events," *JAMA Psychiatry*, Jul. 9, 2014.

Dr. Armon Neel, Jr., "10 drugs that may cause memory loss," *AARP*, Jun. 2015, https://www.aarp.org/health/brain-health/info-05-2013/drugs-that-may-cause-memory-loss.html#quest1

Dr. Armon Neel, Jr., "10 types of meds that can cause insomnia," *AARP*, Apr. 8, 2013, https://www.aarp.org/health/drugs-supplements/info-04-2013/medications-that-can-cause-insomnia.html.

"Lipitor: The Common Drug that Destroys Your Memory," interview of Dr. Duane Graveline with Dr. Joseph Mercola, Feb. 12, 2011, 2011, https://articles.mercola.com/sites/articles/archive/2011/02/12/dr-duane-graveline-on-cholesterol-and-coq10.aspx.

"13 million more Americans would take statins if new guidelines followed: study," *CBS*, Mar. 19, 2014, https://www.cbsnews.com/news/13-million-more-americans-would-take-statins-if-new-guidelines-followed-study/.

David M Diamond and Uffe Ravnskov, "How statistical deception created the appearance that statins are safe and effective in primary and secondary prevention of cardiovascular disease," *Expert Review of Clinical Pharmacology*, Vol 8, No. 2, Feb 12, 2015.

Kelly Brogan, M.D., "Cracking the Cholesterol Myth: How Statins Harm The Body and Mind," *Green Med Info*, Feb 27, 2015.

Part Four:

Ray Sahelian, M.D., *Mind Boosters: A Guide to Natural Supplements that Enhance Your Mind*, (St. Martin's Griffin, Jul. 7, 2000).

Dr. Kelly Brogan, "Why women need to get enough magnesium," *MindBodyGreen*, Nov. 26, 2013.

"Magnesium Deficiency 101," Magnesium Advocacy Group, http://gotmag.org/magnesium-deficiency-101/.

Dr. Jacob Teitelbaum, "Getting a great night's sleep with fibromyalgia, even after you've tried everything," *Intelligent Medicine*, Sept. 23, 2015.

Alan R. Gaby, M.D., "Nutritional treatments for insomnia," *Holistic Primary Care*, Dec. 19, 2011.

Alan R. Gaby, M.D., *Nutritional Medicine*, (2nd ed., 2017).

Tamara Eriksen, ND, "Glycine – Improving Sleep Quality," *Naturopathic Currents*, Apr. 3, 2014.

Part Five:

Dr. Steven Y. Park, *Sleep, Interrupted: A Physician Reveals the #1 Reason Why So Many of Us are Sick and Tired* (Jodev Press, Feb. 9, 2012).

CHAPTER TWO

OPTIMIZE YOUR HORMONES

PART ONE

TUNE UP YOUR HORMONAL SYMPHONY

Right now, a symphony is playing inside your body – a "hormonal symphony" that impacts every cell and function. When your hormonal symphony plays in tune, you feel vibrant and cognitively sharp. When it's off balance, you suffer profoundly. Your energy and memory fade, and you get sick with all kinds of painful problems.

Here are just a few of the common symptoms associated with hormonal imbalance: **depression, anxiety, brain fog, memory loss, exhaustion, insomnia, unexplained weight gain or weight loss, changes in appetite, low libido, infertility, digestive problems, and hair thinning or hair loss.**

By Age 70, Your Youthful Hormones Drop as Much as 90 Percent

"The hormonal symphony means that there are youthful hormones and aging hormones. As we age, our youthful hormones, like **growth hormone, testosterone, estrogen, and thyroid decrease**. By the time you turn 70, they can decrease in some individuals by as much as 90 percent," Dr. Vincent Fortanasce, author of *The Anti-Alzheimer's Prescription,* told me.

"However, the aging hormones – and that is mainly the **cortical steroids** – increase by 60 percent. So at about 50, that's when people really start looking different. And their memory starts to significantly become impaired," he added.

That's why it's crucial for your brain health that you optimize your hormones. By boosting youthful hormones and reducing the aging ones, you'll feel years – maybe decades - younger and sharper.

Tuning Each Instrument in the Hormonal Symphony

Hormones are chemical messengers that help to regulate your metabolism, growth, sexual function, and cognitive function. Each hormone has a vital role to play, and when one hormone blasts too loud in the hormonal symphony or sinks to a whisper, every other hormone is affected.

"Basically, if one hormone is off, it can disrupt all the others," Dr. Shari Caplan, the founder and Medical Director of VitalityMD in Toronto, Canada, told me. "It's important to balance them. When your hormones are restored to optimal levels, you get increased stem cell production for repair and regeneration. And you also have less inflammation."

Each hormone makes an essential contribution to brain health and neurotransmitter function:

- **Testosterone** promotes executive function in the frontal lobe. Both men and women have testosterone, although women have lower quantities.

- **Progesterone** helps to grow new neurons. It binds to the GABA receptor, which helps with sleep, thus acting as a natural tranquilizer.

- **Pregnenolone** influences learning and memory. It's the precursor hormone to numerous other hormones, including testosterone and estrogen.

- **Estrogen** helps produce serotonin, our happy neurotransmitter. It protects the brain against insult and increases nitric oxide, which promotes better blood flow to the brain. Both sexes have estrogen, in differing amounts.

- **DHEA** supports the production of myelin, a protective sheath for nerve cells.

- **T3** is the active thyroid hormone, helping with mood, concentration, and cleaning up brain junk.

Most of the hormones mentioned above work to prevent amyloid plaque deposition, a hallmark of Alzheimer's. They also protect against the loss of brain cells and stimulate the growth of new ones. All hormones are neuroprotective.

Breaking News: Your Brain Makes Hormones, Too

Dr. Caplan explained to me that hormones are made primarily in glands in the body. For instance, the ovaries make estrogen and progesterone, and the adrenals produce cortisol and DHEA.

"However, the newest information is that **the brain has the ability to make hormones, too.** They're called neurosteroids; but if the brain cells are inflamed because of diabetes, toxins, trauma, Alzheimer's, aging, etc., they can't make them."

"So we get a double whammy as we age: our hormones decline in the periphery and also in the brain. That's why it's very important to reduce inflammation and balance hormones by replacing deficient hormones to optimal levels."

From Alcohol to Vitamin Deficiencies: Meet the Hormone Wreckers

Aging isn't the only culprit that disrupts your hormonal symphony. Poor lifestyle choices and other biochemical calamities can take a toll, along with natural stages of the life cycle.

Dr. Pamela Wartian Smith, in her excellent book *What You Must Know About Memory Loss & How You Can Stop It*, names a host of factors that provoke hormonal imbalance, including:

Alcohol abuse, andropause (male menopause), caffeine, chemotherapy, childbirth, endocrine disorders (diseases of the pituitary, thyroid, parathyroid, adrenal, and pancreatic glands), endometriosis, environmental toxins, genetics, head injury, infection, lack of exercise or too much exercise, nutritional deficiencies, obesity, certain pharmaceutical drugs (including antidepressants and birth control pills), perimenopause and menopause, polycystic ovary syndrome (PCOS), poor diet, pregnancy, recreational drug use, stress, and vitamin deficiencies.

Of course, you could have several factors that work together to wreak hormonal havoc. For instance, you may have a poor diet that leads to nutritional deficiencies and obesity; in addition, you may take an antidepressant. Each of these components contributes to your hormonal imbalance and needs to be addressed, in order for you to restore your health.

PART TWO

HOW TO BALANCE AND BOOST YOUR HORMONES

Healthy habits will reduce inflammation, lower aging hormones, and boost youthful hormones. It's time for you to:

Ditch the sugar and eat healthy whole foods. A study found that obese people with elevated insulin levels from sugary food had lower levels of growth hormone, which is crucial for cell growth and regeneration.

Make deep sleep a priority. Your body produces about 75 percent of its growth hormone during the "slow-wave" stages – stages three and four – of deep sleep. As you age, deep sleep markedly decreases, as does nightly secretion of growth hormone critical to brain health. So you need to prioritize good sleep.

Exercise. Recent studies show that exercise improves production of neurotransmitters and neurotrophic factors, thereby boosting new brain cells and connections.

Take control of stress. Stress floods your brain with cortisol, a steroid hormone that shrinks the hippocampus. A fascinating study monitored the cortisol levels of stressed-out caregivers for Alzheimer's patients. After two months of yoga, meditation, and other calming techniques, their cortisol levels had dropped.

Consider taking anti-inflammatory supplements. Dr. Caplan told me that she often uses supplements to reduce inflammation in the brain. Here are some of her favorites:

Omega-3 fatty acids (fish oil or krill oil; vegetarians can take microalgae oil), **curcumin**, **Coenzyme Q10**, and **PQQ** (pyrroloquinoline quinone), a vitamin-like compound that stimulates the mitochondria.

BONUS: If you take CoQ10 and PQQ together, they deliver even greater mitochondrial support.

Find Your Optimal Hormone Levels

Your goal is to optimize your hormones. Like Goldilocks, you want your hormone levels neither too high nor too low, but just right for you.

"When hormones are low, the hippocampus withers and dies. For women, you need to measure their **estrogen and progesterone** levels; and for everybody, their **thyroid, DHEA, and testosterone**," Dr. Daniel Amen, medical director of The Amen Clinics, told me. "And I don't want the levels to be merely normal; I want them optimal."

Getting the right level can be a subtle art, as Dr. Amen explained. "If a male goes too high with testosterone, he'll have a crazy sex drive and no empathy, which is a prescription for divorce. But at the same time, you want it high enough so that you have energy and motivation, and your mood is good and your libido healthy."

Getting your doctor to understand the concept of optimized levels may pose a challenge. "**A lot of people are undertreated**, because a doctor does a blood test and says it's normal," Dr. Jacob Teitelbaum, author of *Real Cause, Real Cure*, told me.

"That diagnosis is based on what's called 'two standard deviations.' They take 100 people; the 95 in the middle are defined as normal, and the highest and lowest two and a half percent are abnormal. But if you're in the normal range, it doesn't mean that you're healthy. You can be at the lowest end of normal and the doctor will say you're fine."

"Apply this to shoe sizes. We take 100 people and get a normal range of sizes 5 through 13. I lose my size 12 shoes and the doctor gives me a size 6. I say to the doctor, 'They don't fit!' He looks at me like I'm crazy and says, "It's size 6. It's normal."

So if most doctors don't know how to get you to optimal levels, what should you do?

Where should you go? And now we've arrived at a key question…

Should You Have Hormone Replacement Therapy?

Hormone Replacement Therapy (HRT) may sound kind of scary, especially if you remember shocking news from 2002: "The National Heart, Lung, and Blood Institute (NHLBI) of the National Institutes of Health (NIH) has stopped early a major clinical trial of the risks and benefits of combined estrogen and progestin in healthy menopausal women due to an increased risk of invasive breast cancer. The large multi-center trial, a component of the Women's Health Initiative, also found increases in coronary disease, stroke, and pulmonary embolism in study participants on estrogen plus progestin compared to women taking placebo pills."

That headline was so frightening that HRT lost favor for years. In fact, controversy continues to swirl around this crucially important topic. In September 2017, a large-scale study of 27,000 women, followed for 18 years, found that women who took hormone replacement therapy for seven years had the same mortality rate as women assigned a placebo.

So should you get Hormone Replacement Therapy or not? I reached out to Dr. Pamela Wartian Smith, founder and Medical Director of the Center for Personalized Medicine, for clarification.

Dr. Smith often uses Hormone Replacement Therapy in her practice with dramatic results. And she personally knows how effective it can be, because it saved her from a terrifying bout of insomnia. At the time, she was working as an Emergency Room physician in Detroit Medical Center. Eleven doctors she consulted could only offer a prescription sleeping pill.

"I'd been to an anti-aging conference in which they discussed the role of progesterone in sleep. I decided to test my progesterone level and discovered that it was zero. So I started taking a low dose of progesterone, and soon I was sleeping fine. That experience led me to shift my career after twenty years in the ER to a specialty in metabolic anti-aging medicine."

Bio-Identical Hormones Versus Synthetic Hormones

Dr. Smith uses **bio-identical hormones** in her practice, not the **synthetic hormones** used in the ill-fated 2002 study. Synthetic hormones are manufactured in a laboratory, and have a different composition than the hormones that they mimic.

Bio-identical hormones, on the other hand, are exactly what they sound like: chemically identical to your body's natural hormones. They are developed from soy or yams infused with enzymes. Their "bio-identical" chemical structure enables your brain to absorb them more readily than synthetic hormones.

Getting a prescription for bio-identical hormones is not like getting a one-size-fits-all prescription for a standard medication. "We give tailor-made prescriptions for each individual patient," Dr. Smith told me. "No two are alike."

If you want to explore getting Hormone Replacement Therapy, Dr. Smith suggests that you find a specialist in metabolic anti-aging medicine. "You should see someone who's fellowship-trained in this field, or better yet has a Master's degree in it."

Dr. Caplan offers some additional advice: "Start on hormonal therapies earlier (around the time of menopause) rather than later to have the best outcome and to lower the risk of cardiovascular disease and events."

PART THREE

WHAT YOU CAN DO; WHAT YOUR DOCTOR CAN DO

"Communication between hormones and the brain is strongly two-way:
The brain produces signals that trigger the release of hormones, and hormones from other parts of the body also influence the brain."

— Dr. Daniel Amen, *Memory Rescue*

WHAT YOU CAN DO

1. **Eat a brain-healthy diet.** Load up on vegetables, high quality protein and healthy fats, as described in the chapter on nutrition.

2. **Get better sleep.** Commit to good sleep hygiene and get help for untreated sleep apnea.

3. **Stress less**. Subdue your brain-corroding cortisol. Listen to music, enjoy your hobbies, breathe deeply, pray, meditate, get massages – whatever soothes your stress.

4. **Exercise in bursts**. High-Intensity Interval Training (HIIT) will stimulate your youthful hormones, while burning fat. Walk, swim, work outside in your garden, and keep moving.

5. **Clean up toxins and infections**. Deal with untreated infections like Lyme Disease and toxic exposures like mold.

6. **Supplement wisely**. Consider trying anti-inflammatory supplements to support hormonal balance.

7. **Find a doctor who specializes in metabolic anti-aging medicine**.

WHAT YOUR DOCTOR CAN DO

1. **Test your hormone levels**. Women need their **estrogen and progesterone** levels tested; everybody needs their **thyroid, DHEA, and testosterone** tested.

2. **Decide on appropriate treatment, or recommend a specialist, such as a metabolic anti-aging specialist.**

3. **Review your medications and suggest supplements**.

4. **Test your hormone levels three months after you begin Hormone Replacement Therapy**. Compare your results with your baseline test, and then test at regular intervals.

NOTES:

Part Two:

R. Lanzi, L. Luzi, et al, "Elevated insulin levels contribute to the reduced growth hormone (GH) response to GH-releasing hormone in obese subjects," *Metabolism*, Vol. 48, No. 9, Sept. 1999.

Rebecca Hardy, "How I lost 12 stone and fathered a child: When chef Tom Kerridge realised he was obese, he devised his very own dynamic diet," *Daily Mail*, Jan. 13, 2017.

"Sleep and Human growth hormone," *Tuck*, May 26, 2017; E. Van Carter and L. Plat, "Physiology of growth hormone secretion during sleep," *Journal of Pediatrics*, Vol. 128, May 1996.

John Cline, Ph.D. "The mysterious benefits of deep sleep," *Psychology Today*, Oct. 11, 2010.

Lila S Chertman, MD, George R Merriam, M.D., et al, "Growth Hormone in Aging," from LJ De Groot, G Chrousos, et al, editors, South Dartmouth (MA); MDText.com, Inc.; 2000-. Updated May 4, 2015.

Sarah DiGuilio, "What Happens In Your Body and Brain During Sleep," NBC News, Sept. 10, 2017.

"While you sleep: sleep isn't a luxury. Skimping on zzz's compromises everything from your immune system to your memory," *NBC News*, Oct. 11, 2017.

Rachel Cooke, "Sleep should be prescribed: what those late nights out could be costing you," *The Guardian*, Sept. 24, 2017.

"Deep Sleep may act as a fountain of youth in old age," *Science News*, Apr. 5, 2017.

Sean Hamilton, "Good doze of medicine: scientists reveal the key to helping you live longer, improve your memory and make you more attractive—and it's sleep," *The Sun*, Oct. 14, 2017.

E. Matta Mello Portugal, E, T. Cevada, et al, "Neuroscience of Exercise: From Neurobiology Mechanisms to Mental Health," *Neuropsychobiology*, Vol. 68, No. 1, March 2013.

Chittaranjan Andrade and Rajiv Radhakrishnan, "The prevention and treatment of cognitive decline and dementia: An overview of recent research on experimental treatments," *Indian Journal of Psychiatry*, Vol. 51, No 1, Jan-Mar. 2009.

M. A. D. Danucalov, E. H. Kozasa, et al, "A Yoga and Compassion Meditation Program Reduces Stress in Familial Caregivers of Alzheimer's Disease Patients," *Evidence-Based Complementary and Alternative Medicine*, Vol. 2013, Article ID 513149.

"NHLBI Stops Trial of Estrogen Plus Progestin Due to Increased Breast Cancer Risk, Lack of Overall Benefit," National Heart, Lunch and Blood Institute, Jul. 9, 2002.

JoAnn E. Manson, MD and Aaron K. Aragaki, MS, et al, "Menopausal Hormone Therapy and Long-term All-Cause and Cause-Specific Mortality," *Journal of the American Medical Association*, Sept. 12, 2017.

Pamela Wartian Smith, *What You Must Know About Memory Loss & How You Can Stop It: A Guide to Proven Techniques and Supplements to Maintain, Strengthen, or Regain Memory*, (Square One, Jan 1, 2014).

CHAPTER THREE

CONQUER YOUR STRESS

PART ONE

WHY YOU MUST TAKE STRESS SERIOUSLY

Stress is chemical warfare against the brain. Left unchecked, it will ravage your brain cells, incite dementia, and eventually kill you.

Dr. Ronald Hoffman, the Medical Director of the Hoffman Center in New York, told me, "Chronic stress, where you're angry, hostile, discouraged and hopeless has a debilitating effect on the whole body. But the brain is particularly vulnerable to that type of stress."

"When you're under stressful circumstances, your learning and memory are impaired. So is your ability to perform and execute. **I think stress is one of the prime factors that affect middle-aged folks who think they may not be recalling well.**"

A big problem with chronic stress is that it becomes a self-perpetuating cycle, in which your brain wires itself to act stressfully. Ken Morehead, an acupuncture orthopedist in North Carolina, told me, "You have to find ways to let stress roll off your shoulders. **If you get in the habit of stress, you're hardwiring neurological pathways that do stress,** and nothing else."

Stress Interferes With Youthful Hormones

Why is stress so dangerous? Perhaps because it disrupts your "hormonal symphony," the complex interplay of hormones that keeps you on track. Dr. Vincent Fortanasce, the author of *The Anti-Alzheimer's Prescription*, told me, "There are youthful hormones that keep us young, strong, and repair the body, such as testosterone, estrogen, and growth hormone."

"On the other side, we have cortisol and cortisone, and glucocorticoid steroids, all of which are stress hormones. And what they do is break down the body."

Stress Shrinks the Hippocampus by 20 Percent – In Just Three Months!

"If a person is under a tremendous amount of stress for three months, we have two NIH studies which show that the hippocampus, the area involved with learning, will decrease in size by 14 to 20 percent in a three-month period. **And that's why stress brings on Alzheimer's and kills – not only the body, but also the brain,**" Dr. Fortanasce said.

Stress Raises Dementia Risk by An Astonishing 65 percent

Consider this Swedish study, which followed 1,415 women, aged 38 to 60, over the course of 35 years. After studying their records, researchers concluded that stress raises dementia risk by a jaw-dropping 65 percent!

That's why it's so vitally important for you to learn how to control stress and build your resilience.

PART TWO

LEARNING TO DEAL WITH STRESS

Some stress is good for us, because humans are not designed to lie in a hammock all day, eating nectar. We thrive on overcoming challenges.

"Everybody is stressed; it's a fact of life. Without stress on our system, nothing happens. **It's our ability to deal with stress that allows us to grow and develop,"** Dr. Allan Warshowsky, an integrative physician in New York, told me.

A busy working mother I know recently described her hectic schedule. I offered sympathy, and she replied, "Yes, but as soon as I head towards home, I can feel my brain changing, getting happy and relaxed because I'm about to see my daughter."

I love the way she worded that. She could *feel her brain changing*, because, in fact, it was. Hormones of happiness were bathing her brain in rejuvenating chemicals, while stress hormones washed away in the tide.

Resilience Keeps You Strong

So how should we deal with stress? How can we move forward through our difficulties calmly and with control? A key concept here is *resilience*, which my dictionary defines as "the capacity to recover from difficulties; toughness."

"Resilience is the ability to take stressful circumstances and surmount them. You put it in the proper context, then move on and transcend the stress," Dr. Hoffman told me. "It's often not possible to change your stressful circumstances, but you can alter the way you respond to them."

Should You Take Tranquilizers?

Let's be candid about what may happen if you go to a doctor and say that you're stressed. Chances are excellent that you'll walk out with a prescription for a benzodiazepine tranquilizer like Xanax or Ativan.

You already know that this type of drug is ripe for abuse, and can lead to physical and psychological dependence. But these medications pose an additional risk: "If you take too many of them, they'll affect your memory. You'll become confused. You may have trouble operating machinery or driving," Dr. Hoffman told me. "These drugs will calm you, but they'll also sedate you."

Is sedation really the best you can hope for? Dr. Hoffman doesn't think so, which is why he likes to use a more holistic or natural approach. His goal is not to tranquilize patients, but to help them feel "**calm, relaxed, and focused.**"

To achieve that goal, Dr. Hoffman sometimes advises his patients to take specific supplements with anti-stress properties. If you're experiencing chronic stress, you may want to try some anti-stress supplements and evaluate their effect.

Of course, you should not go off any medications without your doctor's supervision. And consult your doctor before starting any new supplements.

Four Anti-Stress Supplements That Build Resilience

MAGNESIUM: More than 300 biochemical reactions in your body depend on magnesium, an underappreciated essential mineral. During times of stress, your burn rate of magnesium increases, and you may need to add magnesium supplements to your daily routine.

"My favorite supplement for stress is magnesium," says Dr. Hoffman. "Magnesium is depleted when you're subject to stress, and low levels of magnesium make you jumpy and more irritable. It has a generally relaxing effect on the body, and the vast majority of us don't get enough of it."

Taking magnesium can be a little tricky, because it doesn't easily penetrate the blood-brain barrier. One option is to brew the magnesium-rich banana tea you'll find in the first chapter. You can also add **magnesium mineral drops** to your water; take **magnesium oil footbaths**; soak in **Epsom salt baths**; take a high-quality **magnesium supplement**, or use a **transdermal gel** with magnesium at bedtime.

RHODIOLA ROSEA ("Arctic root" or "golden root"): A wild herb from the high mountains of Asia, rhodiola calms the emotions while stimulating the mind. It's classified as an **adaptogen,** a category of botanical plants that strengthen and balance the body's response to every kind of stress: emotional, physical, and environmental.

Dr. Patricia Gerbarg, a leading expert in natural supplements and co-author of *The Rhodiola Revolution*, told me that she often pairs **schisandra chinensis**, a Chinese medicinal herb, with rhodiola. Some people may experience rhodiola as too stimulating, making them feel slightly jittery; in those cases schisandra can offer a calming balance.

Caution: Rhodiola may not be safe for people with bi-polar disorder.

OMEGA-3 FATTY ACIDS: "In terms of psychology and the brain, the healthiest fat comes from fish," Dr. Hoffman told me. "The omega-3 fatty acids have a very nice effect on the brain, and a stabilizing effect on mood."

"There have been studies of individuals who tried to commit suicide. One group was given fish oil pills and the other was given placebo pills. The group that took the fish oil pills had half the risk for subsequent suicide attempts." (You'll find more information on omega-3 fatty acids in the supplements chapter.)

BIO-STRATH: My personal go-to supplement in times of stress is Bio-Strath, a Swiss herbal tonic brimming with 61 vital nutrients. I learned about it from Dr. Richard Brown, a New York psychopharmacologist and expert on herbal supplements. "It's a good delivery system for B vitamins," he told me. "And doctors who train with me say the most valuable thing they ever learned from me is the importance of B vitamins." I buy mine online; it comes in liquid and tablet form.

PART THREE
SEVEN PROVEN WAYS TO GET CALMER

After speaking to many experts, I've compiled an arsenal of stress-busting techniques. These highly effective tools require no drugs and can help you feel calmer and more in control.

STRESS-BUSTER #1: BREATHE

The hallmark of life is breathing. If you learn just a few simple breathing techniques, you'll always have a fast, non-drug solution to cool down anxiety and lift your mood.

"Studies are revealing that by changing the patterns of breathing it is possible to restore balance to stress response systems, calm an agitated mind, relieve symptoms of anxiety and post-traumatic stress disorder (PTSD), improve physical health and endurance, elevate performance, and enhance relationships," wrote Richard P. Brown, MD and Patricia L. Gerbarg, MD, in *The Healing Power of the Breath*.

A variety of online videos demonstrate simple breathing techniques, such as Belly Breathing, Alternate Nostril Breathing, and Quick Coherent Breathing from HeartMath.com. You can also download an app to guide you, such as Breathe2Relax, BreatheWell, and Paced Breathing.

STRESS-BUSTER #2: MEDITATE

Meditation may sound mystical, but a recent UCLA study discovered a practical benefit: slowing the age-related loss of gray matter in the brain.

Researchers compared brain images of people who habitually meditated and people who did not. And they were surprised by how much more grey matter was preserved in the brains of the meditators. Dr. Florian Kurth, of the UCLA Brain Mapping Center, said they observed "a widespread effect of meditation that encompassed regions throughout the entire brain."

Meditation Encourages a Calm, Cheerful State of Mind

Meditation trains its practitioners to live more "in the moment," through a variety of breathing and visualization techniques. In recent decades, the practice of "mindfulness meditation" has grown more popular to manage stress.

I asked my friend Jill about meditation, because I've noticed how much it helped her. "My life got hectic, dealing with my aging parents," Jill told me. "I couldn't maintain my normal cheerful state, so I went four times to a meditation class."

"I used to get up every morning and start dealing with emails. Now I wake up and meditate for twenty minutes. My mood has really improved and I'm sleeping better."

How To Get Started Meditating

You can take a class; learn from online videos, or try a meditation app. HeadSpace is probably the best known, but others like Calm and Insight Timer have their fans. Each program also has a website for those who prefer apps on their computers.

STRESS-BUSTER #3: ENJOY NATURE

I recently discovered a delightful parody of a pharmaceutical commercial. Instead of hawking a prescription drug, this "commercial" touted the healing powers of nature: "*Tired, irritable, stressed? Try Nature! Side effects may include spontaneous euphoria, taking yourself less seriously, and being in a good mood for no apparent reason.*"

The creators of Nature Rx (www.nature-rx.org) made their spoof to inspire people to get outdoors and reconnect with the natural world. And plenty of studies back them up: nature is good for your physical and cognitive health.

But do you really need studies to tell you how good you feel when you walk in the woods, work in your garden, or skip stones across a lake? Nature Rx is free and waiting to refresh you.

STRESS-BUSTER #4: EXERCISE

Exercise is one of the most powerful stress-busters in the world. In fact, it's so effective that The Anxiety and Depression Association of America says "it's considered vital for mental fitness, and it can reduce stress…Exercise and other physical activity produce endorphins – chemicals in the brain that act as natural painkillers – and also improve the ability to sleep, which in turn reduces stress."

While all forms of exercise are beneficial, some doctors told me that **yoga** and **tai chi** are particularly useful in times of stress.

STRESS-BUSTER #5: EXPLORE THERAPIES LIKE CBT, EMDR, EFT

"I feel so much better," a friend told me, when I bumped into her on the street. "I've been doing Cognitive Behavioral Therapy, and all this baggage I've been carrying around since childhood is finally going away."

COGNITIVE BEHAVIORAL THERAPY (CBT) is usually a short-term treatment that focuses on specific goals. Patient and therapist work together to identify and change negative thoughts that promote self-destructive behavior.

Studies confirm that CBT can effectively treat a range of problems, including sleep disorders, anxiety, depression, substance abuse, eating disorders, and phobias. According to the Mayo Clinic, CBT can help anyone dealing with stressful emotional challenges, such as controlling anger, resolving relationship problems, coping with grief, and overcoming trauma.

CBT offers a more affordable therapy option than open-ended therapy, because it's usually structured for a limited number of sessions.

EYE MOVEMENT DESENSITIZATION AND REPROCESSING THERAPY (EMDR)

Several years ago, I sat next to a woman at a social affair and had a conversation I never forgot. When I learned she was a therapist, I asked if she enjoyed her work. To my surprise, she answered, "I do now. I didn't used to, because I couldn't help people. But now I can, and it's very satisfying."

When I asked what's different now, she answered, "EMDR." She then explained that EMDR (Eye Movement Desensitization and Reprocessing Therapy) is a weird-sounding but amazingly effective treatment for overcoming trauma. In a structured series of sessions, patients recall disturbing memories, while rapidly shifting their eyeballs from side to side.

90 percent of PTSD Victims Healed After 3 Sessions

According to the EMDR Institute, millions of people have been successfully treated, including crime victims, combat veterans, survivors of war, accidents, child abuse, and other traumas.

The Institute's website states, "Twenty positive controlled outcome studies have been done on EMDR. Some of the studies show that 84 percent to 90 percent of single-trauma victims no longer have post-traumatic stress disorder after only three 90-minute sessions."

A Skeptic Becomes a Believer

Rhona Bezonsky, MSW, a psychotherapist in Montreal, told me: "I was initially very skeptical. Even when I applied the technique and saw it working, I was skeptical. I thought my patients would regress and come back. But for the most part, they were basically rehabilitated with relatively brief treatment, compared to other methods."

EMOTIONAL FREEDOM TECHNIQUE (EFT)

It might seem strange to rhythmically tap yourself on acupuncture meridian points while saying positive affirmations. But that's how you perform the Emotional Freedom Technique (EFT), which aims to release negative emotions and unleash blocked energy.

Dr. Joseph Mercola calls EFT "psychological acupressure." He wrote, "more than any traditional or alternative method I have used or researched, EFT works. I have witnessed the results in my patients since deciding to use EFT exclusively in June of 2001."

Gain Control Over Cravings, Fears, and Depression

EFT can help with a wide variety of ailments, including physical pain. You can use it to conquer cravings for food, alcohol, or other unwanted habits; overcome phobias; ease depression or anxiety; and release painful memories.

EFT is free. You don't need a therapist, though you can find one if you prefer. Everything you need to get started is online. On his website, EFT developer Gary Craig offers several instructional videos, including "The EFT Basic Recipe," and "EFT #2, Let's Do It." Other helpful online videos can be found at Tapping.com.

STRESS-BUSTER #6: PRAYER AND FAITH

Our grandparents would not be surprised to learn that prayer is a proven path to de-stressing. But times have changed, and prayer may not come as naturally anymore.

"When I give talks about brain health, I speak about the power of prayer and spirituality," Paul Nussbaum, Ph.D., a clinical neuropsychologist at the University of Pittsburgh School of Medicine, told me. "And afterwards, people will come over to me and whisper, 'Thank you for talking about a Higher Being and prayer.'"

"Prayer is one of the greatest stress reduction techniques," Dr. Pamela Wartian Smith, the founder and Medical Director of the Center for Personalized Medicine, told me. "**Prayer helps you let go and let God – whatever religion you may be.**"

A Sense of Purpose Cuts Your Mortality Risk in Half

People with faith may find it easier to feel a sense of purpose, which energizes and uplifts them. Researchers at Rush University Medical Center studied mortality rates among older adults over a five-year period. They discovered that, "**a person with high purpose in life was about half as likely to die over the follow-up period compared to a person with low purpose.**"

Dr. Nussbaum told me, "I ask people, 'Why are you here? What do you want to do when you wake up in the morning?' Discovering the deep calling inside is powerful medicine."

STRESS-BUSTER #7: PRACTICE GRATITUDE

"Gratitude is the sign of noble souls," said the ancient Greek writer Aesop. It's also the sign of healthier minds and bodies.

"Your brain actually changes when you express and act on your feelings of gratitude. Research has demonstrated that," Dr. David Perlmutter, the author of *Brain Maker*, told me. "I think that gratitude is the antidote to the detrimental effects of stress."

According to a California study of heart attack patients, people with an attitude of gratitude made a better recovery. "It seems that a grateful heart is indeed a more healthy heart, and that gratitude journaling is an easy way to support cardiac health," the study concluded. You can create your own gratitude journal by writing down each day five things that make you feel grateful.

The great religions strive to instill gratefulness through prayers. For instance, Judaism structures one hundred blessings into every day, starting with a prayer of gratitude for waking up. Giving thanks calms our anxieties and elevates awareness of our gifts.

PART FOUR

THE BEST ANTI-STRESS SECRETS OF TOP DOCTORS

I reached out to doctors from a wide range of specialties to learn their best advice on dealing with stress. And I received a wealth of wisdom, which you're about to discover.

PAUL NUSSBAUM, Ph.D., ABPP
STRESS AFFECTS YOUR ABILITY TO RETAIN INFORMATION

"A lot of 50-year-olds come to me thinking they have Alzheimer's. They come in with word-finding problems, distress, sleep problems, memory failures. I'll put them through Hopkins Verbal Learning and other tests, and they'll do just fine."

"So I have to ask them, if the data shows you're in the normal range, why are you in such distress? We tend not to take stress seriously. But it's a very real thing that impacts your ability to retain information."

"The hippocampus of your brain consolidates memory. Right next door is the **amygdala, which triggers the 'fight or flight' response**. When you're getting ready to fight a saber-tooth tiger, the amygdala fires. That activation of the amygdala shuts off the hippocampus, the memory center."

"Prayer and meditation and deep breathing are critically important to settle down the amygdala. Sometimes when I'm upset, I walk around and say to myself, 'Paul, settle your amygdala.' "

RONALD HOFFMAN, M.D.
GET YOUR REPORT CARD ON STRESS

"We measure stress through a saliva test that shows levels of cortisol, **a stress hormone that robs memory, because it shrinks the hippocampus**. We do a lifestyle check and give people a report card on stress."

"When they get their report card, they become more aware of the impact of stress. Eating a healthy diet is important. **Patients with memory issues should keep their blood sugar stable, and eat an anti-inflammatory diet, with healthy omega 3 acids, especially DHEA**."

ALLAN WARSHOWSKY, M.D., F.A.C.O.G., A.B.I.H.M.
COPE WITH STRESS TO GROW AND DEVELOP

"Acute stress response allows us to run away from a rabid dog, then go back to relaxing. But some people keep reliving that rabid dog. That's constant stress. "

"We're trying to understand more about different techniques that help: massage, acupuncture, EMDR (Eye Movement Desensitization Reprocessing). **Whatever will work to keep you in the moment and not worrying about what's coming or fretting about what's past.**"

"Stress affects the brain-adrenal axis. Water-soluble vitamins and magnesium get totally used up by adrenal glands under stress. **Stress twitches are caused by magnesium deficiency.**"

"So add back B vitamins and magnesium and Vitamin C. **Adaptogens such as rhodiola and ginseng will help the body adjust to stress.** Taking these supplements, along with techniques that teach you to stay in the moment and smell the roses – that's how you heal the adrenal glands."

VINCENT FORTANASCE, M.D.
TRY TO ELIMINATE UNCONTROLLED STRESS

"Make a distinction between controlled and uncontrolled stress, and try to eliminate uncontrolled stress as best as you possibly can."

"Uncontrolled stress, for instance, is what's going on in the world. People will watch the news before going to bed and think, 'Oh, isn't it terrible that such and such is happening?' But they have absolutely no control over it. And you can't control your children once they get to a certain age."

"But what can you control? You can control your diet. You can control your exercise. You can control your sleep. You can control your cognitive stimulation. So this is where you should put your energy. Rather than listening to the news while you go home, turn on beautiful music. **Good music will stimulate the good hormones like serotonin, dopamine, growth hormone, and it will keep you youthful.**"

PART FIVE

WHAT YOU CAN DO; WHAT YOUR DOCTOR CAN DO TO HELP

"If you ask me what is the single most important key to longevity, I would have to say it is avoiding worry, stress, and tension. And if you didn't ask me, I'd still have to say it."

— George Burns

WHAT YOU CAN DO

1. **Make managing stress a priority**. Once you commit to it, everything else will follow.

2. **Try starting an anti-stress supplement program, with your doctor's permission.** Pick one supplement and start at a low dose to see how you tolerate it. If you need more support, layer on additional supplements.

3. **Learn breathing techniques**.

4. **Stabilize blood sugar with coconut oil**. Take one spoonful in the morning, one in the afternoon, and one at bedtime.

5. **Exercise**. Build some movement into your schedule every day. Consider trying yoga or tai chi.

6. **Meditate**. Take a class; learn from an online video; meditate with an app.

7. **Spend more time in nature**. Invite a friend for a walk.

8. **Do something you enjoy every day**. Unplug from electronics and engage in something playful or creative.

9. **Connect with other people**. Call a friend. Join a club. Go to church.

10. **If you feel you need it, find a therapist who can help**. Consider some of the therapies discussed here.

11. **Pray**.

WHAT YOUR DOCTOR CAN DO

1. Measure your cortisol with a saliva test.

2. Give you a "Stress Report Card." Based on cortisol levels and other data, your doctor can make an assessment of your body's stress load.

3. Advise on a suitable supplement program. Bring the options from this chapter to your doctor, who may not be aware of them. If your doctor is not receptive, consider finding a holistic doctor to work with you.

4. Review your medications. Your doctor can evaluate if they're causing side effects and other problems.

5. Discuss stress reduction techniques. Recommend tools like breathing, yoga, tai chi, meditation, acupuncture, massage.

6. Recommend a therapist, if appropriate.

NOTES:

Part One:

Lena Johansson, Xinxin Guo, et al., "Midlife psychological stress and risk of dementia: a 35-year longitudinal population study," *Brain*, Vol. 133, No. 8, Aug. 1, 2010.

Jacqueline Sahlberg, "Stress causes brain shrinkage," *Yale Daily News*, Jan. 17, 2012.

Part Three:

Richard P. Brown, MD and Particia L. Gerbarg, MD, *The Healing Power of the Breath: Simple Techniques to Reduce Stress and Anxiety, Enhance Concentration, and Balance Your Emotions* (Shambhala, 2012).

Carolyn Abate, "The Best Meditation Apps of 2017," *HealthLine*, May 19, 2017.

David Carbonell, PhD, "A breathing exercise to calm panic attacks," anxietycoach.com.

"Alternate Nostril Breathing Technique (Nadi Shodhan Pranayama)," www.artofliving.org

"Quick Coherence Technique," https://www.heartmath.com/quick-coherence-technique/.

Mark Wheeler, "Forever young: Meditation might slow the age-related loss of gray matter in the brain, say UCLA researchers," UCLA Newsroom, Feb. 05, 2015. ([Note to Lee: there are good brain images with this article.)

Eileen Luders, Nicolas Cherbuin and Florian Kurth, "Forever Young(er): potential age-defying effects of long-term meditation on gray matter atrophy," *Frontiers in Psychology*, Jan. 21, 2015.

Nature-Rx.org

Adam Alter, "How Nature Resets Our Minds and Bodies," *Atlantic*, Mar 29, 2013, an excerpt from *Drunk Tank Pink: And Other Unexpected Forces That Shape How We Think, Feel, and Behave*, (Penguin Press, March 21, 2013).

"Exercise for stress and anxiety," Anxiety and Depression Association of America, July 2014, https://adaa.org/living-with-anxiety/managing-anxiety/exercise-stress-and-anxiety.

BH Krishna, GS Keerthi, et al, "Association of leukocyte telomere length with oxidative stress in yoga practitioners," *Journal of Clinical and diagnostic Research*, Mar. 2015.

Mayo Clinic Staff, "Cognitive Behavioral Therapy," Mayo Clinic, https://www.mayoclinic.org/tests-procedures/cognitive-behavioral-therapy/about/pac-20384610.

EMDR institute, Inc.

Francine Shapiro, Ph.D., *Getting Past Your Past: Take Control of Your Life with Self-Help Techniques*, (New York: Rodale Books, 2013)

The Gary Craig Official EFT Training Centers

EFT Mercola

"Having A Higher Purpose In Life Reduces Risk Of Death Among Older Adults," *Science Daily*, Jun. 18, 2009.

Patricia Boyle, PhD, Lisa L. Barnes, PhD, Aron S. Buchman, MD, et al, "Purpose in Life Is Associated With Mortality Among Community-Dwelling Older Persons," *Psychosomatic Medicine*: Jun. 2009, Vol. 71, No. 5.

Simone Croezen, Mauricio Avendano, Dr. Frank J. Lenthe, et al., "Social Participation and Depression in Old Age: A Fixed-Effects Analysis in 10 European Countries," American Journal of Epidemiology, Vol. 182, No. 2, Jul. 15, 2015.

James Lake, M.D., "Spirituality and Religion in Mental Health: A Concise Review of the Evidence," *Progressive Psychiatry*, Mar. 2012.

Paul J. Mills, PhD, and Deepak Chopra, MD, et al, "The Role of Gratitude in Spiritual Well-Being in Asymptomatic Heart Failure Patients," Spirituality in Clinical Practice, Jul. 20, 2015.

Li Shanshan, ScD, J. Meir, MD Stampfer, DrPH, David R. Williams, PhD et al, "Association of Religious Service Attendance With Mortality Among Women," *JAMA Internal Medicine, Jun.* 2016.

Honor Whiteman, "Death risk reduced for women who frequently attend religious services," *Medical News Today*, May 16, 2016.

CHAPTER FOUR

EXERCISE YOUR BODY

PART ONE

WHY EXERCISE IS THE SMARTEST MOVE YOU CAN MAKE

Have you ever dreamed of finding the fountain of youth? I just found it for you. It's called exercise. And I can hear you groaning already.

Dr. David Perlmutter, the best-selling author of *Brain Maker*, told me, "Exercise makes you feel good. You develop endorphins, so you enjoy life."

Thousands of studies document exercise's life-changing powers. It protects your cardiovascular system and reduces your risk of diabetes, stroke, and cancer. It strengthens bones and muscles, wards off depression and anxiety, and deepens your sleep.

And if you want to regain your brain, exercise is one of the smartest moves you can make. Physical activity is fabulous for your cognitive powers.

"There's such a push for this or that new proprietary drug, or connecting your brain to a computer to upload information," Dr. Perlmutter told me. "The bottom line is get out and huff and puff a little bit, and you're going to **dramatically improve structurally, what the brain looks like, and functionally, what your brain is able to do.**"

Physical Activity Slashes Dementia Risk by 50%

You may have heard of the famous Framingham Heart Study, which began in 1948 and is still going strong. A recent analysis of Framingham data really grabbed my attention, because it showed stunning news about exercise.

By examining information on 3,700 participants (average age 70), researchers learned that the least physically active people were a whopping **50 percent more likely to develop dementia** during the ten-year follow-up. What spectacular protection those exercisers got!

And a noteworthy British study examined 162 pairs of identical middle-aged female twins. Can you guess the biggest factor that predicted which twin scored higher on brain tests ten years later?

It turned out to be **leg strength**. The identical twins with stronger legs at the start of the study – in other words, the more physically fit ones – outperformed their weaker sisters by an extraordinary 18 percent on memory and cognitive tests ten years later. Not only that, but their brains looked impressively bigger and had fewer empty spaces, too.

"It's compelling to see such differences in cognition and brain structure in identical twins, who had different leg power ten years before. It suggests that simple lifestyle changes to boost our physical activity may help to keep us both mentally and physically healthy," said Dr. Claire Steves, who headed the 2015 study.

"Exercise is All About Love"

Despite all the wonderful studies touting exercise, more than half of Americans don't exercise at all. In fact, many of us spend ten hours a day sitting. And as we get older, we tend to sit longer.

I sympathize, because I can always think of fifty things I'd rather do than exercise. But as I interviewed brain experts, they were so insistent that exercise is crucial I began to pay attention.

Dr. Daniel Amen, the best-selling author of *Memory Rescue*, told me that exercise is "all about love." As the founder of The Amen Clinics, he has amassed the world's largest database of functional brain scans – 125,000 of them – and every day he sees visual evidence of brains, before and after exercise.

"People don't get it," he told me with amused frustration. "They say, 'Oh, I don't want to do this.' And I say, 'Stop being a four year old. This is about adult love. You're going to do the right thing, because you love yourself. You love your wife. You love your children. You love your mission in life. You're doing this because you want to extend your life.'"

Dr. Amen also emphasized to me that he does not want to depend on his children as he ages. And he views exercise as one of the key components to keep him independent.

Now you may already have an exercise routine that you diligently perform. If so, I've leaped out of my chair (good exercise) to give you a standing ovation. But I think you'll still find valuable information in this chapter to keep you motivated and increase the effectiveness of your routine.

As for the rest of us, by reading this we're going to get so pumped about exercise that we can't imagine life without it. We'll even discover the minimum amount we can get away with, just in case we don't completely fall in love with it.

PART TWO
FIVE HUGE WAYS THAT EXERCISE KEEPS YOUR BRAIN YOUNG

When you take a walk, work in your garden, go dancing, lift weights, or do any movement at all, terrific things start happening in your brain. These biochemical changes are the real fountain of youth, because they fight off age-related decline and keep your brain operating at peak efficiency.

Here are five powerful motivators to get you off the couch and into your sneakers.

1. Exercise makes your brain bigger.

"When it comes to your brain, size matters," Dr. Amen told me. "It's the only organ in your body where size really does matter."

If you want a big brain, you'll have to work for it. Starting at age 40, the brain's volume and weight decline by a scary five percent every decade. And after age 70, the shrinkage accelerates.

That's where exercise can save you. "You can increase the size of the brain's memory center and improve memory with just one intervention. And that intervention is exercise," Dr. Perlmutter told me.

A study by Kirk Erickson, Ph.D., a neurocognitive researcher at the University of Pittsburgh, showed that one year of **aerobic exercise training increases the size of the anterior hippocampus** by two percent. And even **low intensity walking** can enlarge your hippocampus, according to a 2014 study of older women.

2. Exercise inspires the growth of new brain cells and connections.

Researchers are discovering that one chemical is crucial for enabling the growth of new brain cells and connections: **BDNF** (brain-derived neurotrophic factor.)

"BDNF is basically growth hormone for the brain. When you have higher levels of BDNF, you're resistant to getting Alzheimer's," Dr. Perlmutter told me. "The most powerful way to change your DNA so that it begins to express BDNF is through exercise. Go out and buy a pair of sneakers. And use them for aerobic exercise."

Let's recap: aerobic exercise boosts BDNF, which promotes the birth of new brain cells and connections. Those new networks make your brain bigger, faster, and more resistant to dementia. All for the price of sneakers!

3. Exercise increases blood flow to the brain.

Vascular dementia is the second most common type of dementia after Alzheimer's. It's caused by impaired blood flow to the brain, a common symptom of aging.

Even seniors who don't have vascular dementia may still feel the nasty effects of too little blood flow: **slow thinking, forgetfulness, dizziness, weakness in the limbs, tremors, getting lost, and not remembering the right word**.

Unfortunately, poor circulation in the brain can precipitate Alzheimer's. Dr. Amen told me, "**Low blood flow is the number one brain imaging predictor of Alzheimer's disease.** What makes us vulnerable to blood flow problems? **Being sedentary**. And exercise is probably the single most powerful thing you can do to keep your hippocampus healthy."

4. Exercise stimulates your mitochondria.

A recent Mayo Clinic study probed how various kinds of exercise impact mitochondria, the energy factories in your cells. Young volunteers (between 18 and 30) who did High Intensity Interval Training (HIIT) showed a **49 percent increase in mitochondrial capacity**. And **older volunteers** (between 65 and 80) experienced a practically miraculous **69 percent increase**!

Isn't it encouraging that you can increase your mitochondrial function by 69 percent – without medication?

5. Exercise boosts "feel good" chemicals, so you ward off anxiety and depression.

Exercise helps you put on a happy face – without the dangers of a prescription "happy pill." The Anxiety and Depression Association of America explains: "According to some studies, regular exercise works as well as medication for some people to reduce symptoms of anxiety and depression, and the effects can be long lasting."

Exercise lifts your mood by boosting two beloved neurotransmitters: **serotonin**, which inspires feelings of calm and optimism and **dopamine**, which spurs learning and motivation. It also elevates **opioids** to help ward off pain and stress. In fact, just one hour of "acute exercise" can positively affect mood and cognitive performance, according to a March 2017 article in *Brain Plasticity*.

PART THREE
HOW TO EXERCISE

Now you know *why* you should exercise. Your next step is to figure out *how* to exercise. What type of exercise should you do? How often should you do it? Do you need to join a gym?

The best way to cut through the confusion is to set two big goals:

GOAL #1: SIT LESS, MOVE MORE. Prolonged sitting slows down your metabolism. And that process leads to all sorts of other problems, even if you regularly work out.

Here's an abbreviated list of what you're likely to suffer, as a result of extended couch potato-itis: diabetes, cancer, cardiovascular disease, obesity, muscle and joint problems, and, of course, cognitive decline. Even if you start the day with a vigorous walk or workout at the gym and then sit for hours, you're still in trouble.

That's why I just invented the Anti-Sitting Society and you're invited to join. Our members break up their sitting time with regular bursts of activity. **We get up once an hour and walk around.** We stand up when we talk on the phone. We lift weights while we binge-watch television. **Our core principle is that we look for ways to be physically active throughout the day**.

GOAL #2: COMMIT TO A BRAIN-BOOSTING EXERCISE ROUTINE. Exercise is the best medicine; so make a plan and stick to it. You can do the minimum, but make sure that you at least do that. And what's the minimum? I'm glad you asked. . .

How Much Exercise Should You Do
(or What's the Least You Can Get Away With)

I asked Dr. Perlmutter for the minimum amount of exercise he recommends: "I think **20 minutes a day** is reasonable. New research is actually indicating closer to 45 minutes to an hour. So that's an investment in the future of your brain."

20 minutes a day doesn't sound too bad, does it? And here's good news from the U.S. Department of Health and Human Services: **"People gain health benefits from as little as 60 minutes of moderate-intensity aerobics per week."**

Dr. Amen told me, "I'm a total believer in, 'What's the easiest way I can get this done?' **So I lift weights for about 35 minutes, twice a week**. And at 63, I'm stronger than I've ever been. And **I walk a lot**, but while I walk, I burst." (Note: I'll explain about Burst exercises – also known as High Intensity Interval Training – in the next section.).

What Type of Exercises Boost Your Brain

Your weekly routine should include **aerobic exercises** to raise your heart rate, as well as **strength exercises** to build your muscles. Both types are proven protectors of the brain.

1. AEROBIC EXERCISES: Running, biking, fast walking, dancing, playing sports, swimming, climbing stairs: all these aerobic activities stimulate the heart to pump faster and deliver oxygen to your muscles.

Moderate aerobic exercise raises your heart rate and makes you sweat, but you can carry on a conversation while you move. **Vigorous aerobic exercise** increases your heart rate so much that you can't talk.

Burst Exercise, also known as **High Intensity Interval Training (HIIT),** is a highly efficient form of aerobics that's gotten popular lately, with good reason. Bursting takes less time than other aerobics, burns more fat, and kickstarts your metabolism.

When you do Bursting, you quickly alternate between full "bursts" of intense activity and periods of much less intense motions. For instance, you may run for one minute, then walk for two minutes; then run for another minute. After fifteen minutes, you've surpassed the health benefits of one hour on the treadmill.

Dr. Amen recommends it: "Rather than just be on a bike for half an hour, it's much better to sprint for 30 to 60 seconds, and then go at a normal pace. Then sprint again for 30 to 60 seconds, and do that four or five times. Your metabolism will go up, and it's also been shown to increase blood flow."

Coordination Exercises will improve your hand-eye cooperation, delivering lots of bonuses to your brain. Dancing, jump rope, and racquet sports enhance coordination, while providing a terrific aerobic workout.

"Coordination exercises boost your cerebellum in the back bottom of your brain, which help turn on your frontal lobe, so your judgment and decision making get better," Dr. Amen told me.

Walking is actually a miracle of exercise efficiency. You can walk briskly for a vigorous aerobic workout (about four miles per hour), walk slower for a moderate aerobic workout, or walk in bursts for a High-Intensity Interval Training workout.

Even a modest amount of daily walking can be a boon to your brain. Dr. Fred Pescatore, a leading integrative physician in New York, recommends daily walks to his patients with cognitive decline.

"A brisk walk without stopping 15 minutes a day will decrease your progression from mild to moderate, and from moderate to major cognitive impairment," Dr. Pescatore told me. "If 15 minutes a day can do that, isn't that something you want to do?"

2. STRENGTH TRAINING: Plan on doing 20 to 30 minutes of strength training two or three times a week. You'll increase muscle mass, improve bone density and reduce your aches and pains. You'll look leaner, reduce your risk of falls, and, of course, boost your cognitive function. That's a pretty big payoff for about an hour a week.

You don't need a gym for strength training; you'll find plenty of options for home or on the move. Use your **body weight** for pushups, pullups, squats, and crunches. You can **lift barbells or dumbbells**, use **resistance bands**, or work on a **weight machine**.

Dr. Vincent Fortanasce, a neurologist and rehabilitation specialist, says that **isometric exercises** are the most powerful brain boosters. To do isometric exercises, hold your muscles in a tense position for ten seconds, release for five seconds, and repeat.

For instance, bring your palms together in a prayer position and tense your muscles as hard as you can. Hold that position for ten seconds and feel the effort in your arms and chest, before you rest for five.

In his excellent book, *The Anti-Alzheimer's Prescription*, Dr. Fortanasce explains that isometric exercise "directly stimulates the brain to produce more growth hormone, testosterone, estrogen, and thyroid hormone – all anabolic hormones or 'the good guys' – to protect the brain." For a video of a complete isometric workout, go to Dr. Fortanasce's website (healthybrainmd. com).

In addition, a good exercise program should also include **STRETCHING** for flexibility and **BALANCE EXERCISES** to prevent falls. One option is **yoga**, which relieves stress, too.

PART FOUR
EASY TIPS TO KEEP YOU ON TRACK

Get up; get moving, and start feeling great. Here are a few practical tips to insure your fitness success.

1. Take "Exercise Snacks"

You might get greater benefits from "exercise snacks" throughout the day than from one long workout. **Prediabetic volunteers who broke their workout into three daily "exercise**

snacks" controlled their blood sugar better than those who performed a long workout. And people with high blood pressure who walked ten minutes three times a day had **better blood pressure** than those who did a single 30-minute walk.

If you really want to do the bare minimum, even **one minute of intense exercise** can help. A McMaster University study showed that people who embedded one minute of "all-out" exercise into an easy 10-minute workout three times a week reaped big rewards. After six weeks, their **endurance, blood pressure, and cellular energy biomarkers** all significantly improved.

Not bad for a mere **three minutes a week** of intense exercise!

2. You're Never Too Old to Start

Listen to 90-year-old Shirley Friedman: "I never had physical training before. I'm a beginner." But then she started regularly working out with Martin Luther King Addo, a former Mr. Ghana bodybuilding champion. Now Shirley reports, "I can walk better and faster, and I don't have that fear of falling." Mary Killoran, 86, also started an exercise routine with Mr. Addo, and she's traded her walker for a cane.

Here's more good news: a study of obese senior citizens who started exercising and added more fruits and vegetables to their diet showed they **improved their physical function, on average, by 21 percent.** Exercise truly can improve your life at any age.

3. Make Exercise Enjoyable

If you don't love exercise, amplify its fun factor. Work out to music you enjoy. Invite a friend to join you. Exercise outside in a beautiful place.

You can also make exercise into a competitive game with activity trackers like a pedometer or workout app. One of my friends recently transformed her body, with help from Fitbit. I'm no longer flustered when she marches around the room, tracking her steps, while we chat.

4. Mix It Up

Don't let boredom stop you from exercising. In fact, you'll get better results by mixing it up. Dr. Pamela Wartian Smith, the author of *What You Must Know About Memory Loss and How You Can Stop It*, works with her patients to create a varied routine.

"One patient and I came up with an exercise plan that she was willing to commit to. Once a week, she walked. One day, she went out square dancing, which she loved. And the other day, she went to the gym for weight training."

5. Avoid Injury

Don't overdo it. Respect your body's limits. After age 50, joint and muscle injuries double every ten years, according to Dr. Fortanasce. For this reason, he also warns seniors not to run. "Running is often dangerous for those over 60," he told me. "It is a cause for knee, ankle, and hip degenerative disease, especially if you are overweight."

And please **make every effort to avoid head injury.** Wear a helmet when you're biking, and take precautions when playing sports. You don't want to suffer from a concussion or head trauma, so play it safe.

6. No Excuses

What if you're plagued with painful joints or other physical problems? Do you get a pass from exercising? No, says Dr. Perlmutter. "I'm in the gym next to people who have terrible knee issues, with multiple operations, and they're on a machine that allows them to become aerobic, based on using their upper extremities."

"Some people are really out of shape. But you could walk from your front door to the mailbox, as a start. There's always a way to do more than you're doing right now."

Of course, you should exercise caution and common sense. **Consult your doctor before starting an exercise program.** If you're 50 or older and have not exercised much, ask if you need a stress test before engaging in physical activity. Begin any new exercise program slowly.

PART FOUR

WHAT YOU CAN DO; WHAT YOUR DOCTOR CAN DO

"Lack of activity destroys the good condition of every human being, while movement and methodical physical exercise save it and preserve it."
— Plato

WHAT YOU CAN DO

1. **Commit to make exercise a regular part of your life**. Write down your reasons for wanting to achieve fitness and regularly review them, if you feel your motivation slacking.

2. **Begin gently and gradually increase your exercise intensity.** Use common sense to avoid injury. Don't push too hard, too fast.

3. **Get an exercise buddy.** Invite a neighbor to join you for a morning walk or yoga class. If you both put it on your calendar, you're more likely to actually do it.

4. **Set an exercise schedule.** Write in your calendar at least three planned exercise sessions per week. For instance: Monday, 5:00 – 6:00 Dance Class; Wednesday 9:00 – 9:30 Walk with Pam; Friday at 1:00 Gym.

5. **Find ways to sneak exercise into your day**. Get off at an earlier bus stop and walk. Forgo the elevator and climb the stairs. Dance while you get dressed.

6. **Find varied exercises to teach your brain to expand.** The richer your exercise routine, the richer your brain neural network. Add a new eye-hand game to the mix.

7. **Improve your posture and breathe deeply.** Good posture and deep breathing are great exercises in their own right.

8. **Don't accept excuses from yourself.** You made an appointment with yourself and you're going to keep it.

WHAT YOUR DOCTOR CAN DO

1. **Give you a green light to start an exercise program**. If you're over 50 and haven't been exercising, your doctor may order a stress test before you start. Make sure to ask if you need one.

2. **Recommend an appropriate exercise routine**. Discuss suitable and varied workouts to increase your strength, flexibility, and endurance.

3. **Help you resolve pain issues, so you can exercise**. Don't let aching hips, knees, neck, or other areas stop you from getting fitter. Work with your doctor, so you can stay active.

4. **Recommend a physical therapist, if that is appropriate**.

NOTES:
Part One:
Zaldy S. Tan, Nicole L. Spartano, et al, "Physical Activity, Brain Volume, and Dementia Risk: The Framingham Study," *Journals of Gerontology Series A Biological Sciences and Medical Sciences*, Vol. 72, No. 6, Jun. 1, 2017.
Claire J. Steves, Mitul M. Mehta, et al. "Kicking Back Cognitive Ageing: Leg Power Predicts Cognitive Ageing after Ten Years in Older Female Twins," *Gerontology*, Vol. 62, No. 2, Feb. 2016.
Press Association, "Strong legs linked to mental ability," *Daily Mail*, Nov. 9, 2015.
Amy Norton, "Study: Americans want to be fit, but don't put in the work," *Health Daily News*, Jun. 20, 2017.

Part Two:

R. Peters, "Ageing and the brain," *Postgraduate Medical Journal*, Vol. 82, No. 964, 2006.

L Svennerholm, K Boström, et al, "Changes in weight and compositions of major membrane components of human brain during the span of adult human life of Swedes," *Acta Neuropathologica*, Oct. 1997.

R. Scahill, C. Frost C, *et al, "A* longitudinal study of brain volume changes in normal ageing using serial registered magnetic resonance imaging," *Archives of Neurology*, Jul. 2003, 200360989–994.

Clifford R. Jack, Jr. M.D., Ronald C. Peterson, M.D., et al, "Rate of medial temporal lobe atrophy in typical aging and Alzheimer's disease," *Neurology*, Oct. 1998.

Kirk I. Erickson, Michelle W. Voss, et al, "Exercise training increases size of hippocampus and improves memory," *Proceedings of the National Academy of Sciences of the U.S.A.*, Vol 108, No. 7, Feb. 15, 2011.

Vijay R. Varma, Yi-Fang Chuang, et. al, "Low-intensity daily walking activity is associated with hippocampal volume in older adults," *Hippocampus*, Vol. 25, No. 5, Dec. 26, 2014.

"About Dementia, Types of Dementia, Vascular Dementia" *Dementia Guide*, last updated Sept. 2, 2017.

Tim Newman, "Exercise prevents cellular aging by boosting mitochondria," *Medical News Today*, Mar. 8, 2017.

Matthew M. Robinson, Surendra Dasari, et al, "Enhanced Protein Translation Underlies Improved Metabolic and Physical Adaptations to Different Exercise Training Modes in Young and Old Humans," *Cell Metabolism*, Vol. 25, No. 3, Mar. 2017.

"Exercise for stress and anxiety," Anxiety and Depression Association of America, Jul. 2014.

Julia C. Basso and Wendy A. Suzuki, "The Effects of Acute Exercise on Mood, Cognition, Neurophysiology, and Neurochemical Pathways: A Review," *Brain Plasticity*, Vol. 2, No. 2, Mar. 28, 2017.

Ana Sandoiu, "How does the brain respond to a single bout of exercise," *Medical News Today*, Jun. 17, 2017.

Part Three:

Marilynn Preston, "If chronic sitting kills, take a stand," *Herald Tribune*, Jan. 20, 2015.

2008 Physical Activity Guidelines for Americans, U.S. Department of Health and Human Services.

Dr. Vincent Fortanasce, *The Anti-Alzheimer's Prescription: The Science-Proven Prevention Plan to Start at Any Age*, (Avery, Aug. 4, 2009).

Mark Rippetoe, "Losing Bodyfat or Gaining Muscle Mass: Which is More Important," *Pajamas Media*, Apr. 9, 2015.

Part Four:

Monique E. Francois, James C. Bald, et al, "'Exercise snacks' before meals: a novel strategy to improve glycaemic control in individuals with insulin resistance," *Diabetologia*, Vol. 57, No. 7, Jul. 2014.

Martin J Gibala, Jonathan P Little, et al, "Physiological adaptations to low-volume, high-intensity interval training in health and disease," *Journal of Physiology*, Vol. 590, No. 5, Mar. 1, 2012.

Emanuel Gomes Ciolac, "High-intensity interval training and hypertension: maximizing the benefits of exercise," *American Journal of Cardiovascular Disease*, Vol. 2, No. 2, May 15, 2012.

Jenna B. Gillen, Michael E. Percival, et al, "Three Minutes of All-Out Intermittent Exercise per Week Increases Skeletal Muscle Oxidative Capacity and Improves Cardiometabolic Health," *PLOS One*, Vol. 9, No. 11, Nov. 2014.

Louie Lazar, "A Chiseled Bodybuilder, Frail Clients and a Fitness Story for the Ages," *New York Times*, Jun. 20, 2014.

D.T. Villareal, S. Chode, et al, "Weight loss, exercise or both and physical function in obese older adults," *The New England Journal of Medicine*, vol. 364 No. 13, Mar. 31, 2011.

Dr. Pamela Wartian Smith, *What You Must Know About Memory Loss and How You Can Stop It, A Guide to Proven Techniques and Supplements to Maintain, Strengthen, or Regain Memory*, (Square One, Jan. 1, 2014).

CHAPTER FIVE

EXERCISE YOUR MIND

PART ONE

NOVELTY AND COMPLEXITY
KEEP YOUR BRAIN HAPPY

"You are never too old to set another goal or to dream a new dream," wrote C.S. Lewis. And that advice turns out to be a perfect prescription for good brain health.

Your brain is wired to need the stimulation of new challenges. When you strive to reach goals that test and excite you, you unleash a cascade of positive biochemical changes in your brain. On the other hand, if you settle into a dull, undemanding routine, your brain starts to shrivel and decay. Or, as Bob Dylan put it, "He not busy being born is busy dying."

Make Your Brain Cells Rejoice

"To build brain resilience, there are two important concepts: **novelty and complexity**," Paul Nussbaum, Ph.D., told me. "If you expose yourself to new and complex experiences, your brain cells will rejoice. **Your dendrites, which are the branches extending from your brain cells, will sprout like a tree. And those branches will connect with other branches.**"

"You want your brain to look like a jungle with lots of connections. If we went into the jungle with a weed whacker, we wouldn't get very far, because there's so much growth there. That's what your brain should look like. If something happens to one section of the brain, there are still lots of other connections."

"I explain this concept to my patients, because it makes it easier to understand why going to a museum or the opera is important," said Dr. Nussbaum, a clinical neuropsychologist at the University of Pittsburgh. "When they realize how these complex tasks help the brain, it becomes personal to them."

What Happy People's Brains Look Like

The growing field of brain imaging draws back the cranial curtain, so we can see what a happy brain looks like. Oxford University scanned the brains of 541 volunteers and created a "connectome," a map of the communication pathways between 200 separate brain regions.

The Daily Mail explained the results: "A strong connectivity pattern that included symmetrical peaks on both sides of the brain in five particular regions was seen as 'positive'. The correlation shows that those with a connectome at one end of the scale score highly on measures typically deemed to be positive, such as vocabulary, memory, life satisfaction, income and years of education."

"Meanwhile, those at the other end of the scale were found to exhibit high scores for traits typically considered negative, such as anger, rule-breaking, substance use and poor sleep quality."

In other words, the people with positive "life satisfaction" had brains that looked like the jungle described by Dr. Nussbaum. They had lived in ways that made their brain cells "rejoice," to use Dr. Nussbaum's memorable phrase, by sprouting reams of active connections.

"The Accountants' Brains Didn't Light Up At All"

Dr. Vincent Fortanasce, the author of *The Anti-Alzheimer's Prescription*, stressed to me the importance of doing novel activities outside of your normal routine. He told me about a study that used functional MRI scans to study brain activity in a group of accountants.

"They were asked to put in numbers using their right hand. And the functional MRI showed that when they put in numbers, their brains didn't light up at all. It was an automatic process that was not a challenge. As soon as the accountants were told: 'Stop using your right hand. Use your left hand,' the whole brain lit up. They were doing something novel."

Dr. Fortanasce explained that when we're children, our brains are in the "sponge stage," sprouting trillions of synapses that connect our brain cells. "That network gives us our intelligence and we develop a propensity for things."

"For instance, if you're in a family that loves music, the areas that have to do with music will be four or five times denser than in someone from a family of handymen. In that family, the part of the brain dealing with construction will be five times denser."

Don't Let Your New Brain Cells Die On The Vine

As it turns out, there's an interesting anatomical explanation of why your brain lights up when it's challenged. In her book *Mindshift*, Barbara Oakley, Ph.D., explains that 1,400 new neurons are born every day in the hippocampus, the brain's short-term memory center.

"But unless the brain continues to encounter novel experiences, many of these new neurons will die off before they mature and hook into the neural network, like vines that languish and die for want of a trellis... Learning is like water and fertilizer that encourage growth of those neural sprouts," Dr. Oakley writes.

This Famous Singer Knows How to Keep His Brain Young

A few years ago, I read a charming interview with Charles Aznavour, the famous French singer-songwriter. He was then 91 and still giving concerts that require great mental and physical exertion.

"If you want to die early, you can be lazy, but if you want to live long, you have to work at it," he explained, noting that he plans to live to 120. Undaunted by 17 surgeries, he exercises every day and stays mentally active. "I read one hour every night and I learn one poem every night," he says. "Right now I am reading three dictionaries — Turkish, Russian and Chinese."

To keep himself energized, Aznavour still writes every day. "My wife, she says, 'Stop working! You are old enough to stop.' I say, 'If I stop, I die.' So she says, 'Please continue!'"

Now that's a great way to approach life - and a great way to stimulate new brain cells with thick jungles of connections.

PART TWO
FIVE WAYS TO BE A BRAIN CHAMPION

When I tell people I'm writing about how to keep your brain active, they often say, "Oh, do crossword puzzles." To which I respond, "If you do crossword puzzles, you'll get good at crossword puzzles. That's not enough."

Basically, you don't get a super-charged brain by living a passive, couch potato life – and then doing puzzles. You get the brain you want by taking a fresh, vigorous approach to life. And, honestly, why wouldn't you want to do that, anyway? Isn't life more fun when you keep the game interesting?

Let's look at some ways to keep your hippocampus blooming with new brain cells and connections.

1. Surprise yourself. Try new things.
Remember Dr. Nussbaum's comments that your brain needs **novelty** and **complexity**? Surprise yourself with new hobbies and activities outside of your comfort zone.

You're a good tennis player…Have you ever played the piano? You make quilts for fun. Could you sell them? You love to read. Could you teach at your local youth center?

Recently, a friend surprised me by raving about dragon boat racing. "I was nervous about trying it, but I'm glad I did. I love being on the river and making new friends."

Well, that activity doesn't float my boat, but I know what does: my new career in music. When I write songs and perform them, I can almost feel my brain lighting up in the most satisfying way. What's new and exciting to you?

2. Redefine what success looks like, so you build a successful brain.

Let's say that you get inspired by this information and decide to try something new: ping pong. You get a friend to play with you – and you're terrible! Which of the following responses do you think works better?

- "I stink at this! I have no hand-eye coordination and me playing ping pong is a joke."

- "Wow, I'm really giving my brain a workout! Good for me for trying something so different!"

Redefine your goal: you're not playing ping pong to seek the world championship. You're playing ping pong to invigorate your brain with a new, complex challenge. Of course, if you keep playing, you might love it. But, whatever happens, *by trying something new, you're already a brain champion.*

3. Become ambidextrous in the brain.

Dr. Fortanasce recommends that you encourage your brain to become ambidextrous. In other words, set up constructive crosstalk between the left and right hemispheres, so both sides become more adept.

Here are some of his techniques, which may feel silly at first, but prove useful:

- Wear your watch on your other wrist. (Bonus Challenge: wear it upside down, too.)

- Brush your teeth with your other hand.

- Switch the hands in which you hold your fork and knife.

- Use both sides of your body more often. Activities like **dancing, knitting, sports, and playing a musical instrument** will engage both sides of your brain. How about learning a few juggling tricks to show off at parties?

4. Try monotasking, not multitasking.

A recent study of the human attention span measured it at eight seconds. Just 17 years ago, a Microsoft study clocked it at 12 seconds. "We've lost a third of our attention span in a very short period of time," Dr. Daniel Amen told me.

Not only are we less focused, we may also feel less calm and happy. Scientists at the University of Sussex found that **people who frequently multitask on different gadgets had less gray matter in the anterior cingulated cortex,** which helps process emotions.

I've got a radical idea for the 21st century: why don't we try doing one thing at a time?

5. Refresh your routine.

Brain cells blossom when you meet new challenges. But what if you're locked into a routine, working the same job with the same people, every day?

Try to energize yourself with little novelties. Maybe you can invite someone different for lunch, or walk another route, or take photos along the way. The point isn't the specifics I just mentioned. The point is that if you try, you can shake up your routine.

Personally, I find inspiration in the story of Natan Scharansky, a human rights advocate in the Soviet Union who was imprisoned for nine years, half of that time in solitary confinement. Forbidden to read or write, Scharansky kept his brain active by playing chess games in his head. His jailers "hoped that I would feel weaker and weaker mentally," he recalled later in Israel, where he served as a Cabinet minister. "Actually, I felt stronger and stronger."

PART THREE
SHARPEN YOUR BRAIN WITH ONLINE TRAINING PROGRAMS

You may have wondered if online brain training programs like Lumosity and BrainHQ are worth your time. Can brain games really make your memory act ten years younger, accelerate your reaction time, and lower your risk of depression?

According to several distinguished doctors I spoke with, the answer is yes. Dr. Dale Bredesen, the eminent author of *The End of Alzheimer's*, incorporates brain training into his anti-Alzheimer's protocol.

And Dr. Norman Doidge, a psychiatrist who's a world-class expert in neuroplasticity, told me, "What has been shown persuasively is that people who are, let's say, 70, who have age-related cognitive decline and do these brain exercises can **start to function the way they did when they were 60 or younger, maybe even 55.**"

A recent study brought great news about the power of brain exercises. 2,802 healthy seniors were tracked over ten years. The seniors who played BrainHQ's computerized brain exercises enjoyed a major reduction in their dementia risk.

"Relatively small amounts of training resulted in a decrease in risk of dementia over the 10-year period of 29 percent," said the study's lead author. "And when we looked at dose-response, we saw that those who trained more got more protective benefit."

Slash Your Car Crash Risk By 48%

Here's an example of brain-training benefits that should grab your attention. Is it worth a few minutes of your day to slash your risk of causing a car crash?

Seniors who did BrainHQ's Double Decision exercise notably expanded their "useful field of view," allowing them to more rapidly process visual information at a single glance. In practical driving terms, that meant they made 38 percent fewer dangerous driving maneuvers, stopped 22 feet sooner when driving 55 miles per hour, kept their license later in life, and cut their at-fault car crash risk by a staggering 48 percent. Yes, the number of accidents they had fell by almost half after their brain training.

An Older Brain Can Do Everything A Young Brain Can Do

Dr. Doidge is a big fan of BrainHQ's program; in fact, he devotes a whole chapter to it in his best-selling book, *The Brain That Changes Itself*. BrainHQ was founded by Michael Merzenich, the renowned neuroscientist, whose many achievements include co-inventing the cochlear implant. **"Everything that you can see happen in a young brain can happen in an older brain,"** Dr. Merzenich told Dr. Doidge.

If you want to try it for yourself, go to BrainHQ's website (www.brainhq.com), where you'll find online exercises that "work out attention, brain speed, memory, people skills, navigation, and intelligence."

"Lumosity Boosted My Confidence"

I asked my friend Freida about her experience with online brain training, and she surprised me with her level of enthusiasm.

"I had serious doubts about my memory," she told me. "I was forgetting how to do things I'd known all my life. The thing that scared me was that I had an MRI, which showed a cloudy area of the brain. They told me I could have early Alzheimer's."

At her doctor's advice, Freida started exercising, incorporating more zinc in her diet, and doing Lumosity to train her brain.

"When I first started Lumosity, I felt so stupid I didn't want to look at my scores. But I've been doing it for a year, and last week, I scored in the 94th percentile in memory. And in problem solving, I'm in the 90th!"

"In real life, I remember better. I can recall people's names and focus on reading again. It's fun and it boosts my confidence."

PART FOUR

WHAT YOU CAN DO;
WHAT YOUR DOCTOR CAN DO

"I am always doing things I can't do. That's how I get to do them."
— Pablo Picasso

WHAT YOU CAN DO

1. **Decide to be a brain champion. Look for novel and complex ways to challenge yourself.** Bonus points if you use both sides of the body, like learning dance steps, knitting, or playing sports.

2. **Consider learning a new language.** Dr. Doidge recommends that seniors take on this challenge to improve and maintain memory. The intense focus required will encourage neuroplasticity.

3. **Stimulate your brain with music.** Learn to play an instrument. Sing in the shower, in the car, in a choir. Dance to your favorite songs.

4. **Think of new ways to expand on activities that you already do.** Can you teach it, sell it, form a club around it, travel to do it in another town?

5. **Consider trying an online brain training program like BrainHQ or Lumosity.** Track your progress and keep setting the bar higher.

WHAT YOUR DOCTOR CAN DO

1. **Give you the go-ahead to take up a new physical activity.** Make sure you get your doctor's approval before hurling yourself into a demanding new physical routine.

2. **Optimize your health so you have the energy to take on new challenges.** Are you too tired to try something new? Work with your doctor to find the underlying causes of your fatigue and recharge your energy.

3. **Suggest possible options for activities and recommend a suitable brain training program.**

NOTES:

Part One:

Mark Prigg, "Intelligent people's brains are wired differently: Researchers say 'smart minds' are more likely to be happy, well educated and earn more," *The Daily Mail*, Sept. 25, 2015.

Barbara Oakley, Ph.D., *Mindshift:Break Through Obstacles to Learning and Discover Your Hidden Potential* (New York: TarcherPerigee, 2017).

Kep Kee Loh, Ryota Kanai, "Higher Media Multi-Tasking Activity Is Associated with Smaller Gray-Matter Density in the Anterior Cingulate Cortex," *PLOS ONE*, Vol. 9, No. 9, Sept. 2014.

Jane Fryer, "'Affairs? I'd rather go to Ikea': He's still crooning at 91 but pint-sized French love god Charles Aznavour admits he prefers shopping in the 'wonderful' Swedish superstore," *The Daily Mail*, Jul. 17, 2015.

Part Two:

"Natan Sharansky: How chess kept one man sane," *BBC Magazine*, Jan. 3, 2014.

Part Three:

Jerri D. Edwards, et al, "Speed of Processing Training Results in Lower Risk of Dementia," Alzheimer's & Dementia: Translational Research and Clinical Interventions; Vol. 3, Issue 4, Nov. 2017.

Norman Doidge, M.D., *The Brain That Changes Itself: Stories of Personal Triumph from the Frontiers of Brain Science* (New York: Penguin Books, 2008).

CHAPTER SIX

NOURISH YOUR BRAIN

PART ONE

EATING THE LOW-CARB, HEALTHY FATS WAY

Nothing is more important for your health than what you eat, and nothing is more confusing. The experts have bombarded us with so much conflicting advice over the years that just choosing what to eat for breakfast can prompt an intense internal debate: Should I or shouldn't I? Is this healthy or poison? Whom do I trust?

Food is fuel, and the quality of fuel in your brain will largely determine your health. When fuel flows in a rich, constant supply, your brain cells will flourish and regenerate. When fuel is lousy and insufficient, your brain cells will die.

And, surprisingly, it turns out that food is information, too. That concept comes from the emerging science of epigenetics, which studies how our choices can actually change our genes.

Let's say you eat a diet of highly refined, processed, sugary foods that are packed with unpronounceable chemicals. Or, to put it another way, you eat the Standard American Diet (SAD). Your food choices will then communicate to your DNA: "Toxins are heading your way! Quick, inflame the brain, to help it cope. And make fat – lots and lots of fat - to capture toxic matter. Begin by fattening the belly!"

Dr. Joseph Maroon, a renowned neurosurgeon and expert on nutrition, told me, "If we eat an inappropriate diet with large quantities of sugar, soft drinks and trans-fatty acids on our French fries, it's going to tell our genes to make inflammatory agents. And inflammation is the common genesis of Alzheimer's, stroke, heart attacks, and damage to our joints and endothelium."

And Dr. Amen imparted this unforgettable warning to me: "If you want to give yourself Alzheimer's disease, follow the Standard American Diet."

When the Experts are Dangerously Wrong

Now you may be one of the millions of people who avoided junk food and tried very hard to eat right. You followed the experts' advice to consume lots of carbohydrates and to avoid fats. After all, you were assured that fats are deadly and that whole grains are the key to good health. There's only one problem with that advice: it's wrong.

A massive international study, published in *The Lancet* in 2017, examined the food intake of 135,000 people in 18 countries over 7.4 years. And, contrary to the experts' recommendations pushed on us for decades, here's what the researchers found: **"Huge diet study shows carbs, not fats are the problem."**

In fact, the so-called PURE study discovered that both saturated and unsaturated fats were associated with a *lower* risk of mortality and stroke. The senior researcher noted that, "saturated fat in moderation actually appears to be good for you." And to think that for years we've been told that fats are nutritional villains out to pillage our health!

"We've eaten fat as a powerful source of calories for a couple of million years. Suddenly, 30 years ago, fat was demonized," Dr. Perlmutter told me.

The facts are indisputable: for decades, public health guidelines instructed Americans to shun fats and cholesterol and to eat carbohydrates. So we cut our fat intake by 25 percent, heaped our plates with refined carbs packed with sugar – and suffered an explosion of bad health.

Half of American adults now have diabetes or prediabetes, and more than two out of three American adults are overweight or obese. Those "diabesity" sufferers may be twice as likely to develop Alzheimer's and dementia.

As for all those warnings about the horrors of cholesterol – oops! In February 2015, the U.S. Dietary Guidelines Advice Committee reversed its longstanding disapproval, writing, **"Cholesterol is not a nutrient of concern for overconsumption."**

Think of all those nourishing eggs you spurned over the years. According to Dr. Walter Willett of the Harvard School of Public Health, "There's never been a single study that showed higher egg consumption is related to higher risk of heart disease."

So are you completely, utterly confused now? *Should* you eat fats? If so, what kind of fats? Should you avoid carbs? *All* carbs? How much protein? What about dairy?

Introducing the Regain Your Brain Food Plan

As a lifelong confused eater myself, I feel enormous satisfaction in offering you a food plan that's backed by impeccable science and inspired by the wisdom of today's most advanced physicians and researchers. And, on a personal note, I love it because it works for me.

This nutritional gift to your brain is called The Regain Your Brain Food Plan. It's a **low-carb, healthy fats, anti-inflammatory, nutrient-dense approach to eating.** And not only will the Regain Your Brain Food Plan invigorate your brain, it will protect your health for the long haul.

I created this food plan based on my extensive interviews with many luminaries of the medical world, including Dr. David Perlmutter, Dr. Daniel Amen, Dr. Dale Bredesen, Dr. Mary Newport, Dr. David Katz, and leading nutritional researcher Dominic D'Agostino, Ph.D. I read dozens of books, pored through the latest research, and combined their findings into an easy-to-understand, easy-to-follow plan.

The Regain Your Brain Food Plan will bestow an abundance of blessings on your health. Here are just a few.

Boost your mitochondria: These powerful energy factories reside in every cell of your body, with a particularly high concentration in the brain. "There are hundreds of mitochondria in each cell, converting oxygen and glucose to energy," Dr. Maroon told me. "Many of the neurodegenerative diseases of aging such as Alzheimer's are related to mitochondrial dysfunction."

That's why a key benefit of The Regain Your Brain Food Plan is its mitochondrial stimulation. According to The Institute for Functional Medicine, "When your mitochondria are working well, they help to reduce fatigue, pain, and cognitive problems, while supporting muscle mass and burning excess fat. Which means that you feel better, think more clearly and have less aches and pains, all while improving your body composition."

Slash your risk of dementia by up to 90 percent: If your current diet is carb-heavy, check out this stunning Mayo Clinic study. For four years, researchers tracked the cognitive status of more than 1,000 seniors, while monitoring their fat, carbohydrate and protein intake.

Here's the jaw-dropping result: **The seniors who ate the most carbohydrates ran an almost 90 percent higher risk of dementia!** And the seniors whose calories came primarily from fat *reduced* their risk of dementia by about 44 percent. Isn't it great to know that by reducing carbs and increasing healthy fats, you can protect your brain?

Promote healthy weight loss: If you want less fat and more muscles, then low-carb, healthy-fat eating is the way to go. A 2014 study by the National Institutes of Health followed 150 people for a year. One group was assigned to limit carbs; another to limit fats. Neither group had calorie restrictions.

So one year later, what was the result? The **low-carb, high-fat eaters weighed eight pounds less** on average than high-carb eaters. They had increased their lean muscle mass and shed significant body fat. And their markers for inflammation and triglycerides had decreased so much they had moved into a lower-risk category for heart attacks.

The high-carb group "actually lost lean muscle mass, which is a bad thing," said Dr. Darius Mazaffarian, the Dean of the Friedman School of Nutrition Science and Policy at Tufts University. "Your balance of lean mass versus fat mass is much more important than weight. And that's a very important finding that shows why the low-carb, high-fat group did so metabolically well."

I love this study is because it's "free-range." People ate what they felt like eating in the real world, without weighing, measuring, and counting calories. After all, you're going to be eating in the real world, too.

Despite all the evidence, the medical establishment still mostly maintains that "fat is bad/ carbs are good." In fact, The American Heart Association recently doubled down on its warnings against saturated fats. But I think when you try the Regain Your Brain Food Plan, you'll see the validity of its science. You'll feel better – and you can't argue with success.

PART TWO
THE REGAIN YOUR BRAIN FOOD PLAN

The Regain Your Brain Food Plan emphasizes **vegetables, healthy fats, and protein**, with carbohydrates added in modest quantities. **You should aim to consume at least 70 percent of your calories from healthy fats.** Keep in mind that fats are high in calories, so you can reach your 70 percent goal without gorging. To ensure nutritional success, follow these five rules.

Rule One: Eat real food.
Nutrition writer Michael Pollan famously advised, "Don't eat anything your great-grandmother wouldn't recognize as food." For example, Great-Grandma might cook mushroom soup, but her batch wouldn't include the xanthan gum, disodium inosinate, soy lecithin, and thiamine mononitrate in a modern can of soup. Keep it real and keep it healthy.

Rule Two: Avoid sugar (including high-fructose corn syrup, dextrose, barley malt, and dozens of other names that don't sound like sugar, but are.)
You've probably noticed that when you eat sugar, it stimulates cravings for more sugar. If you avoid it, you're spared that problem. Consuming sugar is linked to decreased brain volume, Alzheimer's, diabetes, obesity, high blood pressure, and cancer.

In 2016, a shocking 50-year-old secret was revealed: Harvard University scientists on the payroll of the sugar industry had deliberately deceived the public about the dangers of sugar. Instead, they falsely scapegoated saturated fats as a nutritional villain. Their lies greatly influenced governmental guidelines and are a major factor in our current diabesity crisis.

Rule Three: Minimize or eliminate gluten.

Expect happy surprises when you give up gluten. Dr. Benjamin Asher, a leading integrative specialist in New York, told me, "I've had some miraculous results taking people off gluten. People who were terrible snorers and had all kinds of sleep disruptions went off it and got much better."

And Dr. Robert Mathis, a holistic physician in Santa Barbara, California, told me, "After four weeks of not eating gluten, my gluten-sensitive patients tell me, 'I can't believe how much better I feel. My brain fog has cleared and I don't have an upset stomach.' One woman said, 'I took my family off it; now my husband and I are getting along much better and my kids are behaving better, too.'"

Gluten is found in all forms of **wheat,** including **wheat starch, wheat germ, wheat bran, couscous, durum, farino, faro, graham flour, kamut, semolina, and spelt**. Other grains that include gluten are **barley, bulgur, rye, and seitan.**

Gluten has addictive qualities, which may induce cravings, vertigo, and anxiety. If you're highly sensitive to it, you could get celiac disease, vastly increasing your dementia risk. Many processed foods contain gluten, which is a good reason to avoid them.

Rule Four: Maximize your weight loss.

You'll probably shed unwanted pounds on this plan, with increased muscle mass and less fat. If you want to further increase your weight loss, cut back on portion sizes of all food categories except vegetables. Ketosis and intermittent fasting, which you'll learn about in the next section, can also be valuable tools to enhance and maintain your weight loss.

If, despite your best efforts on this plan, your body stubbornly refuses to shed excess weight, other factors could be in play. You might not have enough vitamin D and your hormones may need balancing. The chapter on hormones has more information.

Rule Five: Quality matters. Eat the best food you can.

Organic foods reduce your exposure to toxins and pesticides. So do foods from non-genetically modified (non-GMO) sources. Grass-fed, antibiotic-free, 100 percent organic meat is your healthiest option. So is wild-caught fish, because farmed fish contains toxins like polychlorinated biphenyls (PCBs), pesticides, and antibiotics. As for oils, those that are cold-pressed and minimally refined have the maximum nutritional value.

The predictable downside of higher quality foods is that they're more expensive. Another practical matter is that when you dine out, you may not find them. Do your best to upgrade the overall caliber of your daily foods.

THE FOODS OF THE REGAIN YOUR BRAIN FOOD PLAN

Here's your nutritional bounty for the brain, organized by category. Keep in mind that foods that others thrive on may not work for you. Discover what harmonizes with your body, and go with that.

NON-STARCHY VEGETABLES (five to six servings a day): Organic, non-GMO

Leafy greens: Spinach, kale, lettuce, Swiss chard, collard greens, watercress, parsley, red and green leaf and romaine lettuce, arugula, mustard greens

Cruciferous: Broccoli, cabbage, Brussel sprouts, cauliflower, bok choy, radish, turnip

Various: Asparagus, onion, garlic, shallot, leek, chive, scallions, celery, fennel, mushrooms, artichoke, sprouts, green beans, jicama,

TIP: Eat a rainbow of colors, so you get the full spectrum of phytonutrients. Try to add vegetables to every meal, including raw veggies.

LOW-SUGAR FRUITS: Organic, non-GMO

Various: Avocados, bell peppers, tomatoes, eggplant, pumpkin, cucumbers, squash, zucchini, lemon, and lime

TIP: Avocado is a high fat food, packed with heart-healthy monounsaturated oleic acid. It also contains more potassium than bananas, plenty of fiber, and a wide range of vitamins and minerals.

PROTEIN (serving size about the palm of your hand): Free-range, grass-fed, organically grown animal protein; and wild-caught, low-mercury fish preferred

Fish: Salmon, mackerel, anchovies, sardines, herring, halibut, bass, cod, trout, snapper, sole, grouper, haddock, flounder, mahi mahi; shellfish such as shrimp, lobster, crab, oysters, mussels, clams

Poultry: Whole eggs, chicken, turkey, Cornish hen, duck, pheasant, ostrich, goose

Meat: Beef, bison, lamb, pork, venison and other wild game, liver

TIP: Make sure your first meal of the day includes protein to give you energy. Whole eggs are a great choice: the yolk is packed with omega-3 fatty acids, choline, and other essential nutrients.

TIP: The SMASH fish (salmon, mackerel, anchovies, sardines, herring) are rich in omega-3 fatty acids, which make them excellent brain food.

HEALTHY FATS (minimally refined, cold-pressed, organic, non-GMO):

Cooking oils: coconut oil, extra-virgin olive oil, MCT oil, avocado oil, sesame oil

Salad oils: coconut oil, extra-virgin olive oil, MCT oil, avocado oil, sesame oil, macadamia oil, walnut oil, almond oil, pumpkin seed oil, flaxseed oil

Butters: grass-fed butter, ghee

Nuts and nut butters: pecan, brazil, macadamia, hazelnut, walnut, pine, almond, cashew, pistachio

Seeds: flaxseed, sunflower, chia, pumpkin, sesame

Olives: black, green, Kalamata

Cheese (low-carb cheeses listed first, then in ascending order of carbs): Brie, camembert, muenster, cheddar, gouda, mozzarella, bleu, cream cheese, Swiss, ricotta, cottage, feta

Beverages: Coconut milk, almond milk

TIP: As a source of saturated fat, coconut oil is a champion. And so is its extract, MCT (medium-chain triglyceride) oil. They both metabolize into ketones, a superb brain fuel. Use coconut and MCT oils, separately or together, throughout the day to support brain function. You can add them to coffee and tea.

TIP: Some fats are terrible for you. Avoid trans-fats, the dangerous sludge lurking in processed foods, fast foods, margarine, and commercially baked goods. And keep away from unhealthy oils containing processed polyunsaturated fats: canola, corn, soybean, peanut, and sunflower. On the other hand, extra-virgin olive oil is wonderful, but investigations show that 73 percent of imported "extra-virgin" olive oils are diluted with cheaper oils. American olive oils fare better.

TIP: It's easy to overindulge in cheese, nuts, and seeds. They're delicious, and before you know it, you've eaten far more than you intended. A serving should be about a handful. If you find that you have trouble controlling portion size, or that you're not losing the weight you want to shed, cut out these categories for a while.

CARBOHYDRATES (small amounts once a day, or two or three times a week):

Legumes: lentils, chickpeas, and the universe of beans (kidney, navy, lima, pinto, pink, red, black, etc.)

Non-gluten grains: amaranth, buckwheat, millet, quinoa, rice (brown, white, wild), sorghum, teff, oats (if produced in a facility that's gluten-free)

High-carb vegetables: carrots, parsnips

Fruit (organic, unsweetened, no sugar added): Blueberries, strawberries, raspberries, blackberries, apple, cherries, grapes, mango, pomegranate seeds

TIP: Fruit juice contains high carbs without the fiber, so it sends blood sugar through the roof. And dried fruits are little bombs of carbs and sugars. Avoid them.

BEVERAGES, SPICES, CONDIMENTS:

Beverages (unsweetened, no sugar added): Filtered water, coffee, tea, green tea, kombucha tea, (occasional) one glass of red wine per day for women; two glasses of red wine per day for men

Spices: Sea salt, pepper, cinnamon, sage, paprika, curcumin, oregano, saffron, dill, etc.

Condiments: apple cider vinegar, mustard, horseradish, mayonnaise, hot sauce, tamari, lemon/lime juice

TIP: Spices increase the nutritional density of your food. Use them freely.

OTHER FOODS:

Dairy (in moderate portions): Milk and cream (small amounts for coffee, tea, recipes), full-fat plain Greek yogurt

Fermented foods: Sauerkraut, pickles, pickled fruits and vegetables, kimchi, kefir, coconut kefir

Dark chocolate: One or two squares daily of high quality, organic dark chocolate with 70 percent or higher cocoa content

TIP: Fermented foods teem with probiotics, helping to support a healthy gut.

LET'S PLAY "SPOT THE CARBS"

Which of your breakfast foods was high-carb?

A) French toast

B) Applesauce

C) Orange juice

Answer: All of them.

Which of your lunch foods was high-carb?

A) Lentil soup

B) Carrots

C) Fruit salad

Answer: All of them.

Which of your dinner foods was high-carb?

A) Whole wheat pasta

B) Sweet potato

C) Cookie

Answer: All of them.

As you can see, it's easy to consume lots of carbs throughout the day. But knowledge is power. So choose from the low-carb, brain-boosting foods listed above to avoid carb overload.

PART THREE
FIVE SMART WAYS TO BOOST BRAIN HEALTH

Now that you know which foods to eat, here are five ways to build on the food plan and achieve even greater success.

BRAIN BOOSTER #1: COOK YOUR FOODS "SLOW AND LOW"

The healthiest way to cook food is slowly at a low heat. "I tell my clients think slow and low for brain health," Donna Brown, a clinical nutritionist in Connecticut, told me. "Not high and fast. Instead of grilling a steak, cook beef slowly in a crockpot to maintain nutritional integrity. Even with vegetables, it's better to cook slowly."

Dr. Leo Galland, an integrative medicine specialist in New York, also emphasized the importance of slow, wet cooking. "As soon as you heat oil, you increase the rate at which it oxidizes and breaks down. So cooking at a low heat is best," he said. "When you cook meat, you produce harmful glycated proteins in the meat. The higher the temperature, the more glycation. I'm not saying never charbroil or roast. But if you steam or poach, there's moisture, which keeps the temperature down and decreases the formation of advanced glycation end products."

"Find recipes that allow for wet cooking. Using sauces may help. Cooking things in parchment paper, especially fish, cuts down on the production of advanced glycation end products. This area of research, which is extensive, has been underappreciated, even in the nutritional medical community."

BRAIN BOOSTER #2: PROMOTE HEALTHY GUT BACTERIA

Keeping your gut healthy is essential, because a leaky gut will ooze toxins into the bloodstream and, eventually, the brain. Dr. Perlmutter explained to me the importance of gut bacteria: "It is the job of many of the hundred trillion microbes that live within us to maintain the integrity of the gut lining. When we damage the gut bacteria by our diets, by our usage of medications, then the gut becomes more permeable."

You can enhance your gut bacteria with a **probiotic**. Choose a high-quality supplement to take on an empty stomach, and swap your brand every six months. Dr. Asher told me that, in his experience, probiotics that contain *lactobiacillus rhamnosus* offer the best support for immune function. In addition, a **prebiotic** supplement, such as acacia gum, will provide fiber on which the gut bacteria can feast.

BRAIN BOOSTER #3: USE KETOSIS TO BURN FAT, BUILD MUSCLES

The Regain Your Brain Food Plan should put you in a mild state of ketosis, in which your body burns fat to use as fuel. Doesn't that sound wonderful? Well, it is.

I spoke with the leading researcher of ketogenic nutrition, Dr. Dominic D'Agostino of the University of South Florida, who explained, "When you implement a well-formulated ketogenic diet, you see five things that I think are important for your overall health and protection. Your blood pressure, blood glucose, heart rate, insulin, and C-reactive protein all go down."

Another blessing of ketosis is that it spurs production of ketones, a superfuel that quickly energizes the brain. That's why ketogenic diets are increasingly famous for their beneficial effects on people with cognitive decline and dementia.

Intermittent fasting can boost you to even higher ketogenic levels. (Read about that directly below.) So can consuming coconut oil and its extract, MCT oil. If you have medical issues, work with a health professional to personalize your ketogenic diet and monitor your progress.

BRAIN BOOSTER #4: TRY INTERMITTENT FASTING

For most of human history, we went hungry for long stretches as we scavenged for food. Our bodies are designed to survive and even thrive during periods of fasting. Recently, intermittent fasting has gained popularity for its ability to reduce inflammation, stabilize blood sugar and promote general health.

When you fast, your body gets fuel by burning fat, and that's great news for people who like being sleek and fit. Ordinary diets promote muscle loss, which slows down your metabolism, making it harder to lose weight.

You can try several approaches to intermittent fasting. The most popular is **Restricted Eating Window Fasting**. Confine your eating to a "window" of eight or ten hours, and fast the rest of the time. So, for example, do all your eating between 11 A.M. and 7 P.M. (Feel free to enjoy your morning black coffee anytime you like.) Basically, forgo any after-dinner snacks and skip breakfast. To intensify the fasting effects, shorten your eating time to four hours. For instance, eat one or two small meals between 2 P.M. and 6 P.M.

This approach is highly flexible and you could do it every day, adapting it to your schedule. Many doctors I spoke with recommend doing this type of fasting at least two or three times a week.

Another popular approach is **Alternate Days Fasting**. On your fasting day, eat one small meal (500 calories for women, 600 calories for men). The next day, eat a regular healthy diet. Then switch back to fasting, and so on, until you lose the desired weight.

The 5:2 Fast is another well-loved variation. Five days a week, eat a regular healthy diet; two days a week (let's say Tuesday and Thursday), restrict yourself to 500 calories. Feel free to mix and match any of these approaches to see what works for you. You can even experiment with longer fasts of up to **72 hours**, several times a year, if you're so inclined.

BRAIN BOOSTER #5: APPRECIATE YOUR FOOD

Dr. Allan B. Warshawsky, an integrative physician in Rye, New York told me, "I try to teach my patients the rules of healthy eating. You should separate from your work before you eat. For instance, do belly breathing before a meal."

"Every tradition has a ritual of prayer or lighting candles before meals. These rituals help separate the stress of the day from the holiness of eating. This is not to be taken lightly and should be done with reverence."

"I also teach people how to chew. If you have chronic bloating, reflux, pain, you need to heal your gut. Proper chewing can help. You can do 50 percent of your digestion in your mouth and give your stomach and intestines a break."

"Chew your food until it's turned into a liquid puree. That's about fifty chews per mouthful. Stay in the moment and appreciate what you're eating. People lose weight if they're more satisfied with smaller amounts. And that's what happens if you chew your food till it just slides down."

PART FOUR

WHAT YOU CAN DO; WHAT YOUR DOCTOR CAN DO

"The doctor of the future will give no medicine, but will interest his patients in the care of the human body, in diet, and in the cause and prevention of disease."
— Thomas Edison

WHAT YOU CAN DO

1. **Eat real foods**. Toss those processed, highly refined, sugary products out of your kitchen and stock up with organic, non-GMO healthy fats, produce, and proteins.

2. **Explore new recipes and "wet cooking" techniques**. Learn how to prepare delicious low-carb, healthy-fat meals that you enjoy. Cook "slow and low" and use "wet cooking" techniques to maximize nutritional value.

3. **Drink water, water, water**. Drink a glass of filtered water as soon as you wake up, and stay hydrated consistently throughout the day. "Pre-load" with water before a meal to prevent overeating.

4. **Add small sprinklings of pink Himalayan salt to your food** to insure adequate sodium levels.

5. **Watch your portion size**. Don't overdo the protein, which is easy to do, and keep your carb load very low. If you find yourself overeating nuts and cheese, cut back or avoid them.

6. **Research ketogenic diets for tips and recipes. Use a ketogenic diet app.**

7. **Supplement with probiotics and prebiotics. Magnesium supplements can help to avoid constipation, when you're in ketosis.**

8. **Try intermittent fasting.** Experiment with different schedules and approaches to discover the best way to meet your goals.

9. **Test your ketosis level with strips.** Available in any pharmacy.

10. **Include coconut oil and MCT oil in your daily routine**.

11. **Appreciate your food; chew it slowly, and digest it gently.**

WHAT YOUR DOCTOR CAN DO

1. Take a complete personal history. Consider the possibility of nutritional deficiencies and food allergies, and order appropriate lab tests.

2. Personalize your food plan and suggest supplements.

3. Test your glucose and ketone levels on a regular basis to monitor your progress.

NOTES:

Part One:

Victoria Miller, Bsc. Andrew Mente, PhD, et al, "Fruit, vegetable, and legume intake, and cardiovascular disease and deaths in 18 countries (PURE): a prospective cohort study," Vol. 390, No. 10107, Nov. 4, 2017.

"2015–2020 Dietary Guidelines for Americans," 8th edition, https://health.gov/dietaryguidelines/2015/resources/2015-2020_Dietary_Guidelines.pdf.

Margaret Wente, "A big fat surprise for dietary dogma," *The Globe and Mail*, Mar. 14, 2015, retrievable as of December 2017.

R.O. Roberts, L.A. Roberts, et al, "Relative intake of macronutrients impacts risk of mild cognitive impairment or dementia," *Journal of Alzheimer's Disease*, Vol. 32, No. 2, Jan. 1, 2012.

Lydia Bazzanno, M.D., Ph.D., Tian Hu, M.D. M.S., et al, "Effects of Low-carbohydrate and low-fat diets: a randomized trial," *Annals of Internal Medicine*, Vol. 161, No. 5, Sept. 2, 2014.

Anahad O'Connor, "A call for a low-carb diet that embraces fat," *New York Times*, Sept. 1, 2014, retrievable as of December 2017.

Part Two:

Daniel J. DeNoon, "7 Rules for Eating," www.*WebMD.com*, March 23, 2009, retrievable as of December 2017.

Cristin E. Kearns, DDS, MBA, Laura A. Schmidt, PhD, MSW, MPH, Stanton A. Glantz, PhD, "Sugar Industry and Coronary Heart Disease Research: A Historical Analysis of Internal Industry Documents," *JAMA Internal Medicine*, Vol. 176, No. 11, Nov. 2016.

CHAPTER SEVEN
CLEAN UP TOXINS AND INFECTIONS

PART ONE
CLEAN OUT BIOTOXINS THAT MESS WITH YOUR MIND

Dr. Mary Kay Ross was working as an emergency room physician when her health began to catastrophically fail. She developed thyroid and respiratory problems and a serious autoimmune disease. In vain, she searched for answers from her medical colleagues.

"I've discovered what a poor job traditional medicine does for chronic illness," she told me. "In an effort to find out where my ailments were coming from and what I could do about them, I became involved in functional medicine."

Eventually, Dr. Ross discovered that the source of her medical nightmare was a flourishing infestation of mold right in her home. Today, Dr. Ross is the founder and director of the Institute for Personalized Medicine in Savannah, Georgia. And she uses functional medicine techniques to help patients devastated by mold and other toxins.

Mold is a Leading Cause of Alzheimer's

"Mold can have a very bad effect on your brain. It's a **biotoxin, and we now know that 25 percent of the population has a genetic predisposition to mold or biotoxin susceptibility**," Dr. Ross told me. "Mold, in particular, through breathing in the spores and the mycotoxins, can cause a great deal of inflammation, and can cause Alzheimer's disease in certain patients."

Mold thrives in a wet, humid environment, erupting within 36 hours of a leak. It easily spreads through the HVAC system (heating, ventilation, and air conditioning) and infiltrates furniture and household objects. And once it travels up the nostrils to the brain, it devastates neurons, causing **brain fog, memory loss, insomnia**, and, all too often, **Alzheimer's**.

In fact, Dr. Dale Bredesen, the groundbreaking author of *The End of Alzheimer's*, has coined a new term, **"inhalational Alzheimer's,"** to describe the dementia caused by breathing in mold toxins.

Lyme Disease Infects at Least 300,000 Americans a Year

Alas, mold is not the only biotoxin requiring our constant vigilance. Lyme disease has reached epidemic levels in the United States. The number of cases reported annually has increased nearly 25-fold since national surveillance began in 1982.

The facts about Lyme disease are terrifying, but we need to know them. Lyme infects at least 300,000 Americans a year. Some experts feel that Lyme is vastly under-reported and that the annual number of new cases may reach a million. No accurate test for Lyme currently exists, which is a big problem, considering that most Lyme patients can't recall getting a tick bite or seeing a rash.

More than 40 percent of patients who are treated with 30 days of antibiotics suffer a relapse. And if that news isn't bad enough, here's the kicker: 40 percent of Lyme patients incur long-term health problems. What a nightmare!

Lyme disease is transmitted by a tick infected with Borrelia burgdorferi, a strain of spirochete bacteria. The tick bites an unfortunate human, enabling the bacteria to crawl along the blood vessel walls, spewing toxins. People infected with Lyme can suffer from joint pain, headaches, dizziness, fever, and, most definitely, cognitive decline. 81 percent of adults report memory loss in later stages of the disease. Other common symptoms include loss of concentration, a tendency to get lost, and slower mental processing.

Dr. Amen told me that at Amen Clinics, they have seen hundreds of patients with difficult psychiatric and cognitive problems who turned out to have Lyme disease. When treated, their symptoms significantly improved.

Here's a common scenario: an older patient tells a doctor that he's losing his memory and feels confused. The doctor says he must have Alzheimer's and gives him a prescription. Now, two horrible things have happened. The patient is taking medication for an illness that he doesn't have. And Lyme disease is ravaging his body and brain, untreated.

The singer-songwriter Kris Kristofferson went public with his struggle with Lyme, which doctors had mistakenly diagnosed as Alzheimer's. "He was taking all these medications for things he didn't have, and they all have side effects," his wife said. On some days, Kristofferson was so far gone that he "couldn't even remember what he was doing from one moment to the next."

Eventually, Kristofferson found his way to a doctor associated with Amen Clinics, who diagnosed him with Lyme disease. The doctor treated him with a protocol that includes antibiotics and hyperbaric oxygen. "Now he's back and touring again," Dr. Amen told me. Kristofferson's friend, Chris Gantry, put it more dramatically. "It's like Lazarus coming out of his grave and being born again," he said.

The Red Tide of Deadly Toxins

Biotoxic dangers lurk in the sea, too, in the form of tiny algae called dinoflagellates. Sometimes they erupt into huge algal "blooms," such as the infamous red tide. "When you hear of towns on the ocean having a red tide, there have been episodes where people develop fibromyalgia and chronic fatigue," Dr. Mary Kay Ross told me, adding that algae can release toxic spores in the air.

A 2008 study noted that, "Over the past few decades, the occurrence of harmful algal blooms (HAB) has increased both in frequency and in geographic distribution in many regions of the world." And the Scripps Institute of Oceanography warns that, "If you are on the Gulf coast of Florida and notice asthma-like breathing symptoms, chances are you are experiencing toxicity from a Karenia bloom."

Use the Shoemaker Method to Heal Biotoxic Damage

How can you regain your brain if you're suffering from biotoxic damage? Be encouraged: you can enjoy tremendous healing, but it's essential you fight this battle with the help of an expert physician. Biotoxic damage is complex, and most doctors are not aware of new protocols to maximize recovery.

For instance, one daunting complication is that people with mold problems often suffer from Lyme, as well. "Why do these two illnesses so often coexist?" writes Dr. Lauren Deville, a naturopathic doctor in Arizona. "The closest I've found to a possible explanation is that the biotoxins from one increase the immune system's susceptibility to the biotoxins of the other."

Dr. Ritchie Shoemaker, a recognized pioneer in treatment of biotoxin-related illness, has trained a growing number of physicians in his protocol. You can learn more about his technique in his book *Surviving Mold* and on his website of the same name. (survivingmold.com)

Dr. Mary Kay Ross told me that she employs some of Dr. Shoemaker's techniques, including the use of cholestyramine, a prescription drug which binds to toxins to remove them. "Cholestyramine is an older drug. It's an easy drug to use and not expensive. You can get it from any pharmacy and it helps people regain clarity when they remove the toxins."

In addition to using binders like cholestyramine, Dr. Ross encourages her patients to commit to the brain-healthy living described in detail in this book. She recommends a low-carb/ healthy fat diet, plenty of exercise, online brain exercises, and mindfulness techniques.

She also suggests supplements such as MCT oil, curcumin, and, if necessary, IV treatments with glutathione. And to help patients detox, she recommends an infrared sauna to encourage sweating. "I often find that people who are very toxic don't sweat," she said.

Dr. Ross's first patient with mold was a nurse practitioner whose toxic damage had reduced her hippocampal volume to one percent. The hippocampus is the most important region of the brain for memory. This patient's Montreal Cognitive Assessment score was 10; today, it's up to 22 and she is resuming her regular activities.

But in order to fully recover from mold, you have to leave the toxic environment, which may be your house or apartment. 'That's probably one of the most difficult parts," Dr. Ross said. "It's a very hard thing to come to grips with."

PART TWO

CLEAN UP OTHER TOXINS THAT ATTACK YOUR BRAIN

"Toxins are one of the sleeper causes of dementia," Dr. Amen told me. Could your memory problems be caused by chemicals from your lipstick, cash receipts, or dental fillings? You may be shocked by some of the possible culprits you'll find listed here.

Dr. Amen has discovered that when brains exposed to toxins are examined with SPECT scans, they show a distinctive scalloping pattern that indicates low activity. Cleaning up toxins can invigorate neural action and allow you to enjoy sharper thinking again.

TOXIC TROUBLEMAKERS:

SUBSTANCE ABUSE (Smoking, alcohol, drugs): Cigarettes are toxic to your brain. To cite only one example, a 2015 study published in *Molecular Psychiatry* found that smokers have a measurably thinner cortex than nonsmokers. The cortex is the brain's outer layer of "grey matter" responsible for thinking, language, perceiving and executive function.

Excess alcohol can shrink your brain, too. "Alcohol is not a health food," Dr. Amen told me. "According to a study from Johns Hopkins, people who drink every day have smaller brains. And when it comes to brain, size matters."

Dr. Amen recently published a study in *The Journal of Alzheimer's Disease* that examined **brain scans of 1,000 marijuana smokers**. "Virtually every area of their brain was lower, especially the hippocampus, the area that dies first in Alzheimer's disease. And from being a psychiatrist for 35 years, I know that the most common complaint among pot smokers is poor memory," Dr. Amen said.

Cocaine, methamphetamines, and others drugs are also "toxic to brain function," said Dr. Amen. "You can just see that on the scans. It's clear."

ENVIRONMENTAL HAZARDS: A grisly array of toxins can lurk in your home, workplace and everyday environment, waiting for you to inhale them, smear them on your skin, and eat or drink them.

Your home could contain **chemically laden cleaning products**, personal care items like **health and beauty items, fireplace fumes, painting and solvent fumes**, and **asbestos**. Your kitchen may be stocked with **foods manufactured with plastic equipment** that leaked plasticizers, and infused with **artificial food dyes, preservatives, and sweeteners, MSG, pesticides,** and **herbicides**. And on your way to work, you may breathe **air pollution, car exhaust**, and **gasoline fumes**.

Certain professions may expose you to heightened risks. Dr. Amen told me that almost all the firefighters he treats have toxic-looking brains from exposure to **carbon monoxide** and **fire toxins**. And pilots suffer from the constant impact of **aviation fuel**, which contains **lead**. Workers in manufacturing jobs may be exposed to various **chemicals** and **heavy metals**.

Even your routine trip to the store is fraught with toxic danger. The **cash register receipts** are printed on thermal paper, which contains **bisphenol A,** a carcinogen. And crumpling the receipt (which we instinctively seem to do) intensifies its absorption. In just ten seconds, this carcinogen can be in your system.

Dr. Fred Pescatore, an integrative physician in New York, lamented the toxic nature of our world. "There are phytoestrogens everywhere," he told me. "These are chemicals that mimic estrogen in the body. They're very harmful, especially for women in terms of breast cancer, uterine cancer. But they're in every cleaning supply, every time you get your clothes dry cleaned, every piece of plastic that you sit on."

"When you realize that a baby is born with over 500 chemicals in the umbilical cord, it's amazing. By the time they get to be 70 and 80 years old, they've been bombarded constantly with chemical stress."

HEAVY METALS: **Mercury, aluminum, lead** and other heavy metals can accumulate to dangerous levels, wreaking havoc on the nervous system. Memory loss, confusion, inability to concentrate, and mood disorders can result.

Mercury can leak into the brain from **dental fillings** and from eating **mercury-laden fish** like **shark, swordfish, king mackerel and tilefish**. Aluminum can be found in **cookware, cans, foil, food additives, antiperspirants**, and **infant immunizations**. Lead is no longer allowed in house paint and gasoline for automobiles, but it can still be found in **old toys** and **older homes with older plumbing and pipes**. And if your work involves manufacturing, you may be exposed to heavy metals.

MEDICATIONS AND MEDICAL PROCEDURES: **Chemotherapy, general anesthesia**, and **leaky silicone breast implants** can release toxins that adversely affect the brain. So can many **medications**. **Benzodiazepines** for anxiety or insomnia and **narcotic pain medications** are just two categories of potentially problematic drugs.

To learn more about the cognitive risk of medications, I reached out to Dr. Dale Peterson, a past president of the Oklahoma Academy of Family Physicians, who is at the forefront of exposing iatrogenic illness. MedicineNet.com defines iatrogenic illness as "an illness that is caused by a medication or physician." In other words, it's a medical treatment that makes you sick – the very opposite of the Hippocratic oath, "First, do no harm."

"**Statins** are a real biggie," Dr. Peterson told me. "Statins have horrible side effects, because cholesterol is essential for brain function. **I see a large number of people on statins with memory problems and symptoms related to dementia**. I had a patient who was a Superintendent of Schools. He couldn't remember my name; he was only vaguely aware of where he was. I took him off statins and he had a profound improvement in cognitive function."

"The other big offenders against the brain are **anti-cholinergic drugs**. Many of them are available over-the counter, and people think that if they're OTC, they must be safe. That's far from the truth. It's more of a subtle effect. Someone isn't as sharp as they should be. It's not a full-blown dementia, but it is adversely affecting their ability to put things together and have a smooth, flowing thought process. Most of these drugs will leave fairly quickly from your system. Within two weeks, there should be a significant improvement."

NOTE: I've included an Addendum at the end of this book with a list of medications that can impact memory and cognitive function.

How to Detox Safely

If you suffer from toxic damage, you need to work with an integrative physician to help you safely eliminate the toxins in your system. Your doctor will know how to test for the presence of specific toxins, and which medications and supplements you need. If you have heavy metal toxicity, you may require chelation therapy, in which a chemical solution called EDTA is injected into your bloodstream to bind to the toxins and escort them out.

Operate on two great principles. First, limit your exposure. Second, strengthen your four organs of detoxification.

Limit your toxic exposure: If you currently indulge in substance abuse, there's no time like the present to cut it out. Get help from a support group and from your physician to ease the transition to recovery.

Take an inventory of your household products and personal care products and see if you can swap them for safer versions. Dr. Amen told me that he uses an app called "Think Dirty." "You scan all your products like shampoo and cosmetics and deodorant and so on, and it tells you on a scale of one to ten how toxic it is," he said. Dr. Amen also urges buying organic food to avoid pesticides.

Additionally, you can review your medications with your physician to see if any of them could be having an adverse affect. If your work exposes you to toxins on a regular basis, explore the possibility of realistic adjustments.

Strengthen your four organs of detoxification: the **kidneys, gut, skin, and liver.** Here's Dr. Amen's advice: "Support your kidneys: drink more water. Support your gut: eat more fiber. Support your skin: sweat, either with exercise or taking saunas. A new study from Finland showed people who took the most saunas had the lowest risk of dementia. Support your liver; I like a supplement called N-acteylcysteine (NAC). It helps with detoxification."

"And eat brassicas, which is a new term for me. They're detoxifying vegetables like kale, Brussel sprouts, broccoli, cabbage, and cauliflower. Add a little olive oil with salt, and they taste awesome."

PART THREE

KNOCK OUT INFECTIONS
THAT RAVAGE YOUR BRAIN

Infections can create neural pandemonium, inflaming and poisoning your brain. Whether from a **bacteria, virus, fungus or parasite**, infections must be eliminated if you want to enjoy robust health. The list of grisly intruders includes yeast (Candida), Lyme, toxoplasmosis (a parasite you may pick up from your cat), syphilis, *Helicobacter pylori (h. pylori),* HIV/AIDS, herpes, Epstein-Barr virus, West Nile virus, and cytomegalovirus.

Rampaging infections can harm more than your memory and cognitive powers; they can damage your mental health. Scientists at Johns Hopkins discovered that yeast infections are more prevalent in people with mental illnesses like schizophrenia and bipolar disorder; furthermore, yeast infections in women with mental illnesses are linked to memory problems.

"If you have problems and they're not getting better with simple things, somebody should **do a disease panel** to make sure you're not at war with some invader like toxoplasmosis that comes from cat feces, or Lyme. Herpes is another one. It's very common, and if you have genital herpes, or you have cold sores, that increases your risk of significant memory problems by 20 percent. And that means a third of the population," Dr. Amen told me.

I asked Dr. Jacob Teitelbaum, author of *Real Cause, Real Cure*, what type of infections can spur serious cognitive issues. "The biggies would be **chronic bladder infections** and **chronic sinus** and **candida** problems," he said. He noted that elderly people often don't feel the symptoms of a bladder infection, because their nerves aren't functioning well enough to relay the irritation to the brain. Therefore, they don't get treatment until the infection becomes a rip-roaring disaster.

To prevent a chronic bladder infection, Dr. Teitelbaum suggests taking a supplement called **d-mannose**. "It's over the counter, cheap, safe, benign, and can be taken with any medication. It has no side effects and you can take it every day," he said.

"The other key infection would be candida, which will reflect as **irritable bowel syndrome** and **sinus problems**. Candida is a **yeast infection** that can cause secondary bacterial infections. There's no test for it. So if you find that you have chronic post nasal drip, clearing your throat all the time, and lots of gas, that's a sign of candida."

You'll need to work with a doctor to clear up your infections; this problem is too serious for you to battle alone. Hopefully, you'll find a doctor skilled in integrative medicine who knows safe, effective techniques and can help you strengthen your immune system.

PART FOUR

WHAT YOU CAN DO;
WHAT YOUR DOCTOR CAN DO

"Based on the evidence of tens of thousands of brain scans I have examined, I believe that "infectious disease" will be an important sub-specialty in psychiatry within the next twenty years."

— **Dr. Daniel Amen,** *Memory Rescue*

WHAT YOU CAN DO

1. **Find a good doctor to work with you.** In the Addendum, you'll find information on how to locate a holistic, integrative, or functional medicine specialist near you.

2. **Limit your exposure to toxins.** Eliminate toxin-laden foods, household products, and personal care items that may cause damage.

3. **Drink plenty of water, and make yourself sweat from exercise and saunas.** Sweating is a powerful, natural way to eliminate toxins.

4. **Make extra efforts to eat right, sleep deep and control stress.** Give your body the tools it needs to get stronger.

5. **Consider taking lion's mane**, a powerful mushroom supplement that strengthens the immune system.

WHAT YOUR DOCTOR CAN DO

1. **Test for possible infections and toxic exposures.**

2. **Prescribe appropriate medications and recommend supplements.**

3. **Test your vitamin D and hormonal levels.** Optimizing your hormones will strengthen your capacity to heal.

4. **Monitor your progress and calibrate medications to ensure complete recovery.**

NOTES:

Part One:

Dale E. Bredesen, "Inhalational Alzheimer's disease: an unrecognized – and treatable – epidemic," *Aging*, Vol. 8, No. 2, Feb. 2016.

"A time for Lyme," Aug. 6, 2015, Woods; see also International Lyme and Associated Diseases Society, Quick Facts, http://www.ilads.org/lyme/lyme-quickfacts.php, undated.

Raphael B. Stricker and Lorraine Johnson, "Lyme Disease: Call for a "Manhattan Project" to Combat the Epidemic," *PloS Pathogens*, Vol. 10, No. 1, Jan 2, 2014.

Elizabeth L. Maloney, "The need for clinical judgment in the diagnosis and treatment of Lyme disease," Journal of American Physicians and Surgeons, Vol. 14, No. 3, Fall, 2009, http://www.jpands.org/vol14no3/maloney.pdf.

Mary Brophy Marcus, "Kris Kistofferson's Lyme disease misdiagnosed as Alzheimer's," *CBS News*, Jul. 20, 2016, https://www.cbsnews.com/news/kris-kristofferson-misdiagnosed-alzheimers-has-lyme-disease/.

Da Zhi Wang, "Neurotoxins from marine dinoflagellates: a brief review," *Marine Drugs*, Vol. 6, No. 2, Mar. 9, 2006; "Dinoflagelletes and red tides," Latz Laboratory, Scripps Institution of Oceanography.

Dr. Lauren DeVille, "Lyme disease and mold: they often go together," Jan. 6, 2017, http://www.drlaurendeville.com/articles/lyme-disease-mold/.

Part Two:

 S. Karama and S. Ducharmem, et al, "Cigarette smoking and thinning of the brain's cortex," *Molecular Psychiatry*, Vol. 20, Feb. 10, 2015.

Dr. Daniel G. Amen, Darmal Borhan, et al, "Discriminative Properties of Hippocampal Hypoperfusion in Marijuana Users Compared to Healthy Controls: Implications for Marijuana Administration in Alzheimer's Dementia," *Journal of Alzheimer's Disease*," Vol. 56, No. 1, Jan. 12, 2017.

Part Three:

Emily G Severance, Kristin L Gressitt, et al, "*Candida albicans* exposures, sex specificity and cognitive deficits in schizophrenia and bipolar disorder," the Nature Partner Journal *Schizophrenia*, May 4, 2016.

CHAPTER EIGHT
CONNECT WITH OTHER PEOPLE

PART ONE
GET A "NATURAL HIGH" FROM SOCIAL CONNECTIONS

People need people – for the sake of our health, our happiness, and, yes, for our brains. For millions of years, our ancestors lived in groups in order to increase their odds of survival. With your posse, you might overcome that saber-toothed tiger. Alone, you were lunch.

Our need for other people is hardwired into our bodies, which are designed to reward bonding and punish too much solitude. When we connect with people, we stimulate a rush of "feel good" neurotransmitters like serotonin and dopamine.

Reach Out and Touch Somebody's Hand

"Most people don't realize that reaching across and touching someone immediately stimulates serotonin," Dr. Vincent Fortanasce told me. "Touch is extremely important."

In fact, the "natural high" we get from good relationships is comparable to a marijuana high, without the unhealthy side effects. Dr. Joseph Maroon told me that positive interactions stimulate the endocannabonoid receptors, the same area stimulated by marijuana.

And then there's the "bliss molecule" – anandamide. "That's the body's own intrinsic feel-good chemical and it's rarely discussed," Dr. Maroon said. "Anandamide is what gets people high on THC, the primary psychoactive component in marijuana. We can release it ourselves without pot by focusing on healthy relationships with other people."

Protect Your Brain from Killer Cortisol

Social connections not only promote "good" biochemicals, they also protect us from cortisol, the "bad" stress hormone. "Strong family and social units help control stress, which is a killer," Dr. Maroon said. "Stress increases cortisol, which shrinks the hippocampus and destroys brain cells."

That's why one of the most powerful ways to regain your brain is to expand and deepen your connection to other people. You'll bathe your brain in rejuvenating biochemicals, and protect it from the lethal effects of stress.

If you're not convinced, consider these two California studies. Researchers tracked nearly 7,000 men and women in Alameda County for nine years, beginning in 1965. And they discovered that people who were isolated from others were *three times more like to die* during the course of the study than those with strong social support.

Cut Your Dementia Risk By 50% With Friends and Family

A 2008 study of 2,249 California women discovered that those who had daily contact with friends and family slashed their dementia risk by a phenomenal **50 percent**! Even those who did not speak to others every day still enjoyed a 26 percent lower risk of developing dementia, if they had a large social network.

One more amazing study: in 2011, Rush Alzheimer's Disease Center completed a five year study of older adults. The most socially active seniors showed 70 percent less cognitive decline than the least socially active. *70 percent*! That's a tremendous argument for social activity.

Unfortunately, it's not that easy to make deep connections today, as I'll candidly discuss.

PART TWO
FINDING CONNECTIONS IN THE MODERN WORLD

Does this sound like your life? You wake up in a family home teeming with children, parents, and grandparents. You spend the morning tending the garden with your spouse; then visit your neighbors for a leisurely lunch. At night, you play dominoes with friends; on Sunday, your family walks to church.

That's how life is lived in Ikaria, Greece, where more centenarians can be found than almost anywhere on earth. On this "island where people forget to die," residents have half the rate of heart disease of Americans and **almost no dementia**. One out of three Ikarians makes it to their nineties, and their lives are filled with contentment, friends and family. As the doctor in Ikaria explained, "It's not a 'me' place, it's an 'us' place."

In the Blue Zones, People Live to 100

Ikaria is one of five so-called "Blue Zones" around the world, the areas where people live the longest. Identified by author Dan Buettner, the Blue Zones share some important characteristics, including a culture that forges strong personal connections.

"They're put together the same way as the rest of us. It's not like they're made of better stuff," Dr. David Katz told me, when I asked why Blue Zones residents routinely live to be 100 without dementia. "The answer is lifestyle."

"They live in cultures where it's normal to eat a wholesome diet, to get routine physical activity, to get enough sleep, not be stressed out. And, in addition, **to have good, supportive, strong interactions with one another, that sense of community**."

Dr. Katz, the Director of the Yale University Prevention Research Center, believes that the Blue Zones have lessons for the rest of us. "*You've got to prioritize relationships*," he said. "That's really the important step."

In Recent Decades, Inviting Friends Over Decreased by 45 Percent

I find it ironic that just as we're getting more evidence of our need for social connections, our world is growing more disengaged. A book published in 2000, *Bowling Alone,* got lots of attention for pointing out that most Americans no longer participated in community groups, and personal bonds were weakening.

According to author Robert Putnam, in the last quarter of the 20th century, American attendance at club meetings went down by 58 percent. Family dinners declined by 33 percent, and inviting friends to one's home decreased by 45 percent.

Americans were "bowling alone:" still bowling, but no longer in leagues, whose rosters had declined by a staggering 40 percent. Putnam worried that Americans were losing the "sturdy norms of reciprocity," those social ties that foster trust and support.

Almost two decades after *Bowling Alone* was published, people are more alone than ever. Our digital buddies often take pride of place over face-to-face relationships. The trend seems to be accelerating: I'm stunned when I walk the streets of New York, where I live, by the number of people with phone in hand, head down, oblivious to their surroundings.

The Isolation of Aging

Getting older can be isolating, too. You may retire and miss out on the daily interactions of work. People you love may move or pass away. Physical limitations can keep you housebound.

"What occurs in individuals who age? Their physical contact decreases almost 100 percent," Dr. Fortanasce told me. "In fact, many people will say that the only time they have any physical contact is when they shake hands with people in church."

Having an active social life definitely takes effort, especially when you're older. But the rewards are worth it. In the words of Helen Keller, "Walking with a friend in the dark is better than walking alone in the light."

PART THREE
CREATE YOUR OWN BLUE ZONE

In the Blue Zones, social connections come naturally. People eat healthy meals together, take walks together, and laugh and pray together. As a result, they constantly reinforce each other's good habits.

Why not try to create your own mini-Blue Zone? Reach out and create a group of people who support the very best in each other. Here are some ideas:

1. Volunteer. Become a docent at the local museum; serve at a soup kitchen. Your years of wisdom can help others, and you'll meet other volunteers.

2. Set up regular dates for meeting people. Fill your calendar with ongoing weekly appointments: Monday is poker night; Tuesday, volunteer at church; Wednesday, take an exercise class, etc. You'll always have something to look forward to and opportunities to mingle with good people.

3. Call friends and family frequently. I know of a local church where the elders have a buddy system. Every morning, they call to check on one another's needs and lend support to get through the day.

4. Take a class. Learn something new and meet people with similar interests. You can find classes at many nearby institutions; your local college may even allow you to audit for free.

5. Join a church or other religious community. Practicing your faith in community is one of the healthiest activities possible. In fact, a European study showed that people who joined a religious group scored higher for "sustained happiness" than those involved in any other social activity.

6. Connect with purpose on social media. Dr. Dale Bredesen, author of *The End of Alzheimer's*, told me about an exciting online support community at ApoE4.info, where people with the genetic marker for Alzheimer's share information and advice. "Social networking is the key to a world without dementia," he said.

Speaking personally, I've seen the power of social networking on our *Awakening from Alzheimer's* Facebook page. We find strength and support from people we've never met who share our deepest concerns.

PART FOUR

WHAT YOU CAN DO;
WHAT YOUR DOCTOR CAN DO TO HELP

"No man is an island entire of itself;
every man is a piece of the continent, a part of the main."

— John Donne

WHAT YOU CAN DO

1. **Explore opportunities to connect in your community**. Check out local organizations where you can volunteer, take classes, or join a group.

2. **Invite your friends to a weekly potluck dinner. Join a book group. Set up a morning walk with your neighbors.**

3. **Get active in your church**.

4. **Increase activities and conversations with your family.**

WHAT YOUR DOCTOR CAN DO

1. **Suggest suitable activities and local resources.**

2. **Recommend a therapist if anxiety or depression are keeping you from socializing.**

NOTES:

Part One:

Lisa F. Berkman and S. Leonard Syme, "Social Networks, Host Resistance, and Mortality: a Nine-year Follow-up Study of Alameda County Residents," *American Journal of Epidemiology*, Vol. 109, No. 2, Feb. 1, 1979.

Valerie Crooks, James Lubben, et al, "Social network, cognitive function, and dementia incidence among elderly women," *American Journal of Public Health*, Vol. 98, No. 7, Jul. 2008.

Bryan D. James, Robert S. Wilson, et al, "Late-Life Social Activity and Cognitive Decline in Old Age," *Journal of the International Neuropsychological Society*, Vol. 17, No. 6, Apr. 8, 2011.

Part Two:

Dan Buettner, "The Island where people forget to die," *New York Times*, Oct. 24, 2012.

Robert Putnam, *Bowling Alone: The Collapse and Revival of American Community*, (New York: Simon & Schuster, 2000).

Part Three:

Olivia Blair, "Going to church 'has a positive long-term effect on mental health for the elderly'," *The Independent*, Aug. 7, 2015.

"Attending church is the key to good mental health among older Europeans," The London School of Economics and Politics, Aug. 4, 2015.

Part Four:

William J. Chopik, "Associations among relational values, support, health, and well-being across the adult lifespan," *Personal Relationships*, Vol. 24, No. 2, April 19, 2017.

CHAPTER NINE

STABILIZE YOUR BLOOD SUGAR

PART ONE

WHY BLOOD SUGAR MATTERS

I recently attended a lecture by a Silicon Valley health guru. "Wanna see something cool?" he said, pointing to his armband. "That's my blood sugar count. Now I instantly know how my blood sugar reacts to every food I eat."

Tracking blood sugar is a hot new Silicon Valley trend, even for people who don't have diabetes. High-tech workers need to operate at peak efficiency, and they know that stable blood sugar levels promote a clear mind and steady energy levels.

Moreover, the biggest tech companies are developing blood sugar monitors for a distressingly huge market. Some **86 million Americans now have pre-diabetes** and **30 million have full-blown diabetes: that's half of American adults**. "What we're seeing at the level of the entire population is a massive prevalence of insulin resistance," Dr. David Katz told me.

Insulin resistance is essentially pre-diabetes. It's a condition that occurs when your cells simply refuse to "open their doors" to the massive amount of sugar in your blood.

Diabetes Raises Your Alzheimer's Risk by 65 Percent

Do you have diabetes or pre-diabetes? If you think you don't, are you sure? You may want to reconsider your answer. According to the Centers for Disease Control and Prevention, 90 percent of American adults with pre-diabetes don't know they have it. And that goes for 25 percent of diabetics, too.

What a dangerous situation! Diabetes hugely raises your risk of heart disease, stroke, blindness, kidney failure, amputations – and, yes, Alzheimer's. The linkage between diabetes and Alzheimer's is overwhelming.

For instance, a study of 824 Catholic clergy showed diabetics run a **65 percent higher risk** of Alzheimer's. And Minnesota researchers found that **81 percent of the Alzheimer's patients they studied had either type 2 diabetes or pre-diabetes**. In fact, Dr. Mary Newport, a Florida neonatologist, told me, "**Alzheimer's disease is a type of diabetes of the brain**."

Even if your blood sugar doesn't rise to diabetic levels, you're still not in the clear. "We found a steadily increasing risk [for dementia] associated with ever-higher blood glucose levels, even in people who didn't have diabetes," said the author of a 2013 study in *New England Journal of Medicine*.

Now for the Good News: You Can Change Your Destiny

That's why it's so important to stabilize your blood sugar. Not only will you enjoy greater mental clarity and physical energy, you'll protect your brain for the long haul.

And here's the good news: you *can* do it. 95 percent of diabetes cases are type 2, which means they were caused by lousy lifestyle choices. Change your habits and you can change your destiny. "I tell my diabetic patients: you ate your way into the situation; you can eat your way out of it," Dr. Fred Pescatore, a New York integrative physician, told me.

If you're 60 or over, all you have to do is lose five to ten percent of your weight to cut your diabetes risk by a phenomenal *71 percent*. So if you weigh 160 pounds and you lose at least eight pounds, you're much likelier to enjoy a longer, healthier life. And at any age, if you lose five to ten percent of your weight, you cut your risk of type 2 diabetes by roughly 58 percent.

"We know that 95 percent of the time, insulin resistance and type 2 diabetes – the metabolic syndrome – are preventable by **eating well, being active, and controlling weight**," Dr. Katz told me. Just **the simple act of walking twenty minutes a day** can lower your risk of type 2 diabetes by 30 percent, according to a huge analysis of 301,221 people.

In fact, it turns out that our grandparents' wisdom about taking a stroll after dinner was right on the money. A Mayo Clinic study found that walking after meals significantly lowered glucose levels in both diabetics and non-diabetics alike. "Minimal activity sustained for 30 minutes (walking 0.7 miles in 33 minutes) lowers post-meal glucose concentrations. Such activity has little or no risk for almost everybody," wrote the study's lead author.

PART TWO

BREAKING THE DIABETES CYCLE

Here's how you give yourself diabetes. You eat high-carb, sugary junk food, which sends your blood sugar skyrocketing. Your cells need blood sugar (also known as glucose) to supply them with energy, but they can't handle too much all at once.

Faced with this huge surge of blood sugar, your pancreas frantically churns out insulin. Think of insulin as an escort for blood sugar, chaperoning it into the cells. By pumping out insulin, your pancreas is attempting to quickly hustle the glucose out of your bloodstream and into its cellular destination.

But as your blood sugar levels crash, your energy crashes, too. You feel tired, listless, and adrift in a brain fog. You're much too exhausted to get off the couch and exercise. So what's going to make you feel good again? Sugar! And so the whole rotten cycle begins again.

Frankly, you're not helped by the junk food industry, which specifically engineers its products to make them addictive. "How did junk become a food group?" Dr. Katz asked me. "Michael Moss, a Pulitzer Prize-winning investigative journalist, tells us that all the big food companies hire whole teams of scientists and give them functional MRI machines and marching orders to design food we can't stop eating. They call it 'the bliss point.' We're telling people, 'Eat well,' but then we have teams of scientists designing food to sabotage that effort."

How to Make Yourself Stupid

Eventually, if you keep on starving your body of proper nutrients, while force-feeding it junk, some predictable disasters unfold.

1) You become overweight or even obese. Excess blood sugar has to go somewhere, and, unfortunately, it goes into your cells as fat. As your waist and other regions expand, your heart, liver, and kidneys also get fat, reducing their ability to function.

2) You develop insulin resistance. Take pity on your poor pancreas, which is constantly kicked into overdrive by your lousy food choices. As it pumps out insulin to deal with excess blood sugar, it confronts a new problem: insulin resistance. Basically, your cells get tired of having to deal with an oversupply of insulin and go on strike. Their refusal to accept insulin means that blood sugar levels keep rising and cells don't get their necessary fuel. A horrible cascade of deterioration ensues.

3) You become one more statistic in the epidemic of "diabesity" – a deadly combination of diabetes and obesity. Research from the Harvard School of Public Health revealed that "being even slightly overweight increased diabetes risk five times and being seriously obese increased it 60 times." Now you've got a potentially fatal "spare tire" around your middle, high blood pressure, high blood sugar, high cholesterol, raging inflammation, mitochondrial dysfunction, and problems with blood clotting.

Plus, you're making yourself stupid. Dr. Amen warned me that "diabesity" shrinks the brain. "I published two studies that showed as your weight goes up, the actual physical size and function of your brain goes down. That's 'dinosaur syndrome' – big body, little brain."

Change Your Health Habits; Change Your Destiny

But if that's your story so far, remember: it doesn't have to be your destiny. You *can* break free to a healthier future by making better choices.

1) Ditch the sugar; eat healthy fats. "You've got to get the food right, because that's how you get diabesity under control," Dr. Amen said. "Basically, it's kill the sugar before it kills you. And kill the foods that turn to sugar – bread, pasta, potatoes, and rice – because they're high glycemic. The real weapons of mass destruction are highly-processed, pesticide-sprayed, high glycemic, low fiber, food-like substances stored in plasticized containers."

Luckily, if you follow The Regain Your Brain Food Plan, you're already on the fast track to better health. You're eating high quality protein, vegetables, and generous amounts of healthy fats. Dr. Dale Bredesen, who made history as the first person to document Alzheimer's reversal, told me, "Fundamentally, you want to convert the system from a carbohydrate-based system to a lipid-based system, so you really want to go towards good fats."

2) Exercise and stay physically active. "I've heard many times from my patients over the years that they don't have time to exercise," Dr. Katz told me. "And my answer has always been the same: 'That's interesting. I don't have time *not* to.' In order to maintain my energy, my enthusiasm, and, frankly, my level of cognitive function, I've got to exercise."

There's no way around it: exercise is essential to combating diabetes. Get in the habit of exercising every day, and remember to regularly enjoy a pleasant walk after a meal. Not only will your blood sugar levels improve, you'll also feel healthier and happier.

3) Get a good night's sleep. What a vicious circle: if you don't sleep well, you increase your risk of diabetes; and if you have diabetes, you probably don't sleep well. That's because your kidneys try to get rid of high blood sugar by urinating. So you wake up frequently to go to the bathroom, disrupting your sleep.

Of course, when you're exhausted from not sleeping, you may try to rouse yourself by eating sugar. And the whole destructive cycle begins again, as the junk food sends your blood sugar skyrocketing.

A big reward of eating better and exercising is that your sleep will probably improve, too. Make good sleep a priority. You'll find it easier to make good choices about food and to motivate yourself to exercise when you're strengthened by a good night's sleep.

Supplements That Help Stabilize Blood Sugar

You may decide to try some supplements to help you control high blood sugar. I asked Dr. Pamela Wartian Smith for her recommendations, and here's what she told me:

ALPHA-LIPOIC ACID: "Many times, if you have a problem with blood sugar, from 300 to 400 mg a day of alpha-lipoic acid can help lower blood sugar and make insulin work better in the body. In fact, if people are already on medication and we start alpha-lipoic acid, sometimes people need less medicine. And alpha-lipoic acid is also very good to help prevent and treat neuropathy, which is the numbness and tingling that some people get when they have diabetes."

BERBERINE: "One of my very favorites is berberine. It's a fabulous anti-inflammatory. Studies have shown it can lower cholesterol and blood sugar in many people. So if you have a cholesterol and blood sugar problem, you can actually get a two-for-one with berberine."

CHROMIUM: "Chromium is a mineral that can decrease sugar cravings. It helps build muscle. When we're healthier, we need just a little bit of chromium. But if blood sugar is awry, or starting to, then we use a bigger dose."

PART THREE

WHAT YOU CAN DO;
WHAT YOUR DOCTOR CAN DO

"The connections among high blood sugar, insulin resistance, diabetes, obesity, and risk for brain disorders are irrefutable."

— Dr. David Perlmutter

1. **Eat a good healthy diet, low on carbs, and rich in healthy fats.** Throw out the sugar and processed food. Load up on fresh vegetables, high quality protein, and healthy fats like coconut oil, olive oil, and avocados.

2. **Lose weight if overweight, and maintain a healthy weight.** Make the commitment to feel better right now and support your long-term health.

3. **Avoid late night eating when your body is more insulin resistant.** Try to go for at least twelve hours after dinner before you eat again. However, you may find a teaspoon of coconut oil at night helps to stop late night cravings.

4. **Exercise regularly and walk after meals.** Physical activity every day will help to control your blood sugar. Get your doctor's permission to exercise more vigorously, so you don't

unduly strain your heart. If you're overweight, just start with walking and gradually build up speed.

5. **Take appropriate supplements.** Discuss your supplement plan with your doctor.

6. **Make good sleep a priority.** Seven to eight hours of deep sleep every night will promote healthy blood sugar levels and bring multiple health benefits.

WHAT YOUR DOCTOR CAN DO

1. **Give you an annual test for pre-diabetes, starting when you turn 45.** If you have a family history of diabetes or a risk factor like obesity, your doctor should start annual tests sooner.

2. **Educate you on how to monitor blood sugar levels.** Knowing how to track your fluctuations will help you stay on target.

3. **Help you choose the appropriate level of exercise.** If you're overweight and sedentary, you don't want to strain your heart. Your doctor can assess the right exercise plan for you.

4. **Discuss appropriate medication and supplements**. As you adjust your eating and exercise habits, you may be able to reduce or even eliminate medications.

5. **Refer you to specialists.** If necessary, your doctor can recommend an eye doctor, cardiologist, nephrologist, and other specialists who can treat problems created by unhealthy blood sugar levels.

NOTES:

Part One:

Christina Farr, "Some Silicon Valley techies are now obsessively tracking their blood sugar – and they don't have diabetes," CNBC, May 15, 2017, retrievable as of December 2017.

Christina Farr, "Apple CEO Tim Cook test-drove a device that tracks his blood sugar, hinting at Apple's interest in the space," *CNBC*, May 18, 2017, retrievable as of December 2017.

"New CDC report: More than 100 million Americans have diabetes or prediabetes," Centers for Disease Control and Prevention, Jul. 18, 2017.

Zoe Arvanitakis, MD, Robert S. Wilson, PhD, et al, "Diabetes Mellitus and Risk of Alzheimer Disease and Decline in Cognitive Function," *Arch. Neurol*, Vol. 61, No. 5, May 2004.

Juliette Janson, Thomas Laedtke, et al, "Increased Risk of Type 2 Diabetes in Alzheimer Disease," Diabetes, Vol. 53, Feb. 2004.

Paul K. Crane, M.D., M.P.H., Rod Walker, M.S , et al, "Glucose Levels and Risk of Dementia," *New England Journal of Medicine*, Aug. 8, 2013.

"Diabetes: Working to Reverse the US Epidemic At A Glance 2016," Chronic Disease Prevention and Health Promotion, CDC, last updated Jul. 25, 2016.

"Diabetes Prevention Program (DPP)," National Institute of Health, U.S. Department of Health and Human Services, undated; "Diabetes Prevention Program (DPP)," National Diabetes Information Clearinghouse, U.S. Department of Health and Human Services, NIH Publication No. 09–5099 October 2008.

Christie Y. Jeon, R. Peter Lokken, et al, "Physical Activity of Moderate Intensity and Risk of Type 2 Diabetes: a systematic review," *Diabetes Care*, Vol. 30, No. 3, Mar. 2007.

"Walking after eating lowers glucose in healthy people and diabetes patients," *Diabetes in Control*, Aug. 31, 2012.

Diane Fennel, "Walking significantly reduces after-meal glucose," *Diabetes Self-Management*, Sept. 14, 2012.

Part Two:

Amy Hess-Fischl MS, RD, LDN, BC-ADM, CDE, "What is insulin," *Endocrine Web*, last updated 4/7/2017, retrievable as of December 2017.

Alvin Powell, "Obesity? Diabetes? We've been set up," *Harvard Gazette*, Mar. 7, 2012.

Denise Mann, "The Sleep-Diabetes Connection: Not sleeping? Check your blood sugar levels," www. WebMD.com, Jan. 19, 2010.

CHAPTER TEN

TAKE SOME SUPPLEMENTS

PART ONE

FIVE ALL-STAR SUPPLEMENTS TO SUPPORT BRAIN HEALTH

When I visit the homes of the eminent doctors I interview, I try to peek at their kitchen counter. Usually, I'm greeted by the sight of at least a dozen supplement bottles. As a matter of fact, that's what my counter looks like, too.

You should get most of your nutrition from your food. And if you follow the Regain Your Brain Food Plan, you will. But the leading doctors I know all believe in taking supplements, too. These safe, natural additions to your daily routine can fortify your brain and prevent heartache down the road.

You may already be taking **a high quality multi-vitamin**; if not, that's an excellent place to start. But what else should you take? I know from readers' comments (and my own experience) that dealing with supplements can be a bit overwhelming. Which ones? What brands? How big a dose? Are they safe with medications?

So I've tried to keep it simple. Out of the abundance of supplements that doctors have recommended, I selected five all-stars for your daily routine. Think of them as your basic supplement wardrobe, equivalent to having a navy blazer and pair of jeans.

You'll note that I recommended other supplements in previous sections, such as **magnesium** for stress, and **alpha-lipoic acid** and **berberine** for blood sugar. Those supplements and many others can work wonders, and I encourage you to consider taking them. You're certainly not limited to the five mentioned here.

Check for contraindications and, of course, speak to your doctor or pharmacist about concerns. In fact, you should always check with your doctor before taking supplements. And now, let me introduce you to…

Five Superb Supplements for Brain Support

SUPPLEMENT ONE: FISH OIL (OMEGA-3 FATTY ACIDS)

Almost every doctor I interviewed chose fish oil as a must-have supplement, especially for people who don't eat fish at least twice a week. Fish oil is rich in omega-3 fatty acids, giving it magnificent anti-inflammatory powers.

Dr. Amen told me. "We did a study of 200 consecutive patients at the Amen Clinics; **95% of them had low levels of Omega-3 fatty acids**. If you have low omega-3's, you often have high inflammation."

Recently, Dr. Amen published a study that showed people with low omega-3 levels have a smaller hippocampus, the crucial brain region where Alzheimer's begins. He also noted that if you suffer from **depression** or other mental health issues, fish oil is a powerful asset.

And here's good news for vegetarians: You can take **microalgae oil** to get your omega-3 supply.

DOSAGE: Dr. Vincent Fortanasce recommends taking 1,000 mg of fish oil twice daily. Your doctor may suggest a different dosage.

CAUTION: People who take blood thinner medications, including aspirin, should be aware that fish oil can affect the clotting ability of blood platelets. Discuss the situation with your doctor.

SUPPLEMENT TWO: CoQ10 (COENZYME Q10)

Coenzyme Q10 is like a spark plug, igniting energy in every cell of your body. A powerful antioxidant, CoQ10 stimulates the mitochondria to produce more energy, and protects the brain from free radical damage. In fact, a Japanese study found that seniors with higher levels of CoQ10 had significantly less dementia.

I'm curious: did your doctor ever give you this **important warning?** If you take **statins** or other common medications, you're compromising your ability to process CoQ10. **Antidepressants, antipsychotic drugs, blood pressure-lowering drugs, cholesterol-lowering drugs, and anti-diabetic drugs** all lower CoQ10 levels.

And there's only one way to boost your CoQ10 levels: with supplements. "It doesn't occur naturally in food. You can't eat your way into CoQ10," Dr. Smith told me.

I recommended CoQ10 to my friend Elizabeth, and here's what she wrote me: "It was so surprising to me that when I started to take CoQ10, I began to feel the way I did when I was younger – that feeling of get up and go. I feel healthier and more buoyant."

CoQ10 in the form of **ubiquinol** is easier to absorb. Ubiquinol is more expensive than CoQ10, but you'll probably need less of it, because of its superior absorption rate.

DOSAGE: Dr. Fortanasce recommends a range of 300 – 1200 mg, depending on your needs.

BONUS: Taking CoQ10 with **PQQ (pyrroloquinoline quinone)** can amplify its power.

SUPPLEMENT THREE: VITAMIN D3

If you're lucky enough to spend your days outside, you may have healthy levels of vitamin D. But most of us are stuck indoors, which is why 75 percent of American teens and adults are deficient in vitamin D3, according to a 2009 article in *Scientific American.*

Despite its name, vitamin D, "the sunshine vitamin," is actually a hormone that positively influences 3,000 genes in your body. "Vitamin D3 is an essential item in terms of neuro-protection, as well as endothelial protection," Dr. Maroon told me. "Endothelial deterioration leads to heart disease and strokes."

Without sufficient vitamin D, you grow more vulnerable to Alzheimer's. A study of 858 older adults published in *Archives of Internal Medicine* found that people with the lowest vitamin D levels were 60 percent more likely to exhibit signs of general cognitive decline. Another study found that the cognitive ability of seniors with low vitamin D declined twice as fast as those with adequate levels.

Dr. Amen got a wonderful surprise by boosting his vitamin D: he dropped 20 pounds. "I tried to lose weight in every way you can imagine. When vitamin D is low, the hormone leptin that tells your brain you're not hungry doesn't work. When I started on vitamin D, my appetite went away."

DOSAGE: Dr. Amen recommends that you measure and optimize your vitamin D3 level. Normal is between 30 and 100; optimal is between 50 and 100. If you live where the sun isn't out for a long time, you probably need **5000 units of vitamin D3 a day**.

BONUS: VITAMIN K2 taken in conjunction with vitamin D3 can increase its effectiveness.

SUPPLEMENT FOUR: CURCUMIN

Curcumin gives curry dishes their gorgeous yellow color. It's the active component in the spice turmeric, and its widespread use in Indian cooking may explain why India has one of the lowest dementia rates in the world.

"If you're going to do something for Alzheimer's prevention, take curcumin," Dr. Jacob Teitelbaum told me. "It's probably the premiere herb for reducing the risk of Alzheimer's."

Curcumin has been shown to reduce inflammation, clear away brain plaque, and protect mitochondria. It can significantly ease joint pain, energize the digestive and immune system, and promote healthy cholesterol levels.

CAUTION: Despite curcumin's glorious qualities, it's notoriously difficult for the body to absorb. Brands vary in their ability to deliver curcumin to the bloodstream, so make sure to find one of high quality. Some brands combine curcumin with piperine, the bioactive compound in black pepper, to increase its absorbability. If you buy a better brand, you'll need a lower dose.

People who take a blood thinner should consult their doctor before taking curcumin. Also, curcumin is not recommended for people with gallbladder or bile duct problems, or who have a tendency to develop kidney stones.

BONUS: Curcumin works better in tandem with **vitamin D3**.

SUPPLEMENT FIVE: B VITAMINS

B vitamins are spectacularly necessary for brain function. Among other benefits, they lower homocysteine levels, preventing this potentially dangerous amino acid from causing inflammation, hardening of the arteries and blood clots.

Consider this study of people who had taken the Scottish Mental Surveys of 1932 and 1947, which measured childhood intelligence. When researchers tested them as older adults, they found the most mentally sharp responders had the *highest* levels of B vitamins and *lowest* levels of homocysteine.

Vitamin B12 deficiency is extremely common among people suffering from memory loss and dementia. And since it's difficult to obtain B12 from food, you most likely will need a supplement. Other B vitamins are equally important, albeit in different ways.

Now I want to ask the same question I asked about CoQ10: Has your doctor ever warned you that taking medications can interfere with your metabolism of B vitamins?

Check to see if you take any of these B-depleting drugs: **aspirin; antibiotics for chronic urinary tract infections; antacid and stomach acid suppressors; anti-diabetic drugs; asthma drugs; blood pressure-lowering drugs; anti-convulsant drugs; cholesterol-lowering drugs; estrogens; estrogen substitutes; anti-Parkinson's drugs; nonsteroidal anti-inflammatory drugs (NSAIDS); and corticosteroids anti-inflammatory drugs.**

If you do, you probably should take daily B vitamin supplements. You should also **ask your doctor to regularly check your homocysteine levels.** Make sure you have an optimal amount of all your crucial B vitamins. In addition to **vitamins B6, B9 (folate) and B12**, you need **vitamin B1 (thiamine), vitamin B6 (pyridoxine) and vitamin B3 (niacinamide).**

DOSAGE: Take a B-complex vitamin twice daily, according to product instructions. Your doctor may prefer for you to take specific vitamin B supplements. For instance, you may be advised to receive a temporary series of vitamin B12 injections, if your levels are critically low.

CAUTION: Work with your doctor to achieve optimal levels and to ensure that your B vitamins are in balance with each other.

PART TWO

WHAT YOU CAN DO;
WHAT YOUR DOCTOR CAN DO

"Clearly, it is important that you supplement your diet with certain nutrients in order to allow your mind to be the best that it can be."

— Dr. Pamela Wartian Smith,
What You Must Know About Memory Loss and How You Can Stop It

WHAT YOU CAN DO

REMINDER: Always consult with your health care practitioner before you start your supplement program.

1. **Pick one supplement to start. Begin at a low dose and build up**. Take it for at least a week before adding another, so you can judge its effects.

2. **Choose a high quality brand.** Pharmaceutical grade supplements meet the highest standards, but are more expensive. If you can't afford them, look for supplements that contain no preservatives or artificial coloring, and are natural, not synthetic.

3. **Try to find smaller capsules for easier swallowing.** Fish oil can come in large capsules; if swallowing is a problem, look for smaller pills. Other tips for smooth swallowing: put pills in applesauce or yogurt. Coat them with a small amount of olive oil. Swallow with a denser fluid like milk, instead of water.

4. **Observe how you're reacting to your supplements, and adjust accordingly.**

WHAT YOUR DOCTOR CAN DO

1. Measure your levels of vitamins D3, B12 and other essentials to assess your optimal dosage.

2. Advise about appropriate supplements for your specific health situation.

3. If all goes well, work with you to cut back on your medications or even eliminate them, if appropriate.

NOTES:

Part One:

Dr. Daniel Amen and William S. Harris, PhD., et al, "Quantitative Erythrocyte Omega-3 EPA Plus DHA Levels Are Related to Higher Regional Cerebral Blood Flow on Brain SPECT," *The Journal of Alzheimer's Disease,* Vol. 58, No. 4, Jun. 2017.

"Can Omega-3 Help Prevent Alzheimer's Disease? Brain SPECT Imaging Shows Possible Link," *Journal of Alzheimer's Disease* Content, May 19, 2017.

K. Yamagishi, A. Ikeda, el al, "Serum coenzyme Q10 and risk of disabling dementia: the Circulatory Risk in Communities Study (CIRCS)," *Atherosclerosis*, Vol. 237, No. 2, Dec. 2014.

Jordan Lite, "Vitamin D deficiency soars in the U.S., study says," *Scientific American*, Mar. 23, 2009.

DJ Llewellyn, IA Lang, et al, "Vitamin D and risk of cognitive decline in elderly persons," *Archives of Internal Medicine*, Vol 170, No. 10, Jul. 12, 2010.

Joshua W. Miller, PhD, Danielle J. Harvey, PhD, et al, "Vitamin D Status and Rates of Cognitive Decline in a Multiethnic Cohort of Older Adults," *Journal of American Medical Association, Neurology*, Vol. 72, No. 11, Nov. 2015.

L Zhang, M Fiala, et al, "Curcuminoids enhance amyloid -beta uptake by macrophages of Alzheimer's disease patients," *Journal of Alzheimer's Disease*, Vol. 10, No. 1, Sept. 2006.

RB Mythri, B Jagatha, et al, "Mitochondrial complex I inhibition in Parkinson's disease: how can curcumin protect mitochondria," *Antioxidants and Redox Signaling*, Vol. 9, No. 3, *Mar.* 2007.

S. Daniel S, JL Limson, et al, "Through metal binding, curcumin protects against lead- and cadmium-induced lipid peroxidation in rat brain homogenates and against lead-induced tissue damage in rat brain," *Journal of Inorganic Biochemistry*, Vol. 98, No. 2, Feb. 2004.

"The Impact of Childhood Intelligence on Later Life: Following Up the Scottish Mental Surveys of 1932 and 1947," *Journal of Personality and Social Psychology*, Vol. 86, No. 1, 2004.

CONCLUSION

FIVE CASE STUDIES

CASE STUDY ONE:
SALLY TOOK FOUR HOURS TO GO FOUR BLOCKS

Sally had an 8 A.M. doctor's appointment, but she didn't show up for it till noon. For four hours, she had been driving around, trying to figure out how to find the office of Dr. Pamela Wartian Smith – which was four blocks from her home.

Sally was 67 when she finally found her way to Dr. Smith, the Founder and Medical Director of the Center for Personalized Medicine in Grosse Pointe, Michigan. "We started working on different things because cognitive decline frequently is multi-factorial, meaning there are a number of reasons why people may have cognitive decline," Dr. Smith told me.

"Hers was stress, because her husband had died, so she was grieving. She wasn't as nutritionally sound as she could be. She wasn't exercising. She was waking up four or five times a night. We measured her thyroid. It was not optimal. Blood sugar was already starting to decline."

"Her female hormones were not perfect, and her hormone pregnenolone, which is the hormone of memory, was unmeasurable. The lowest they can measure is five, and she was at less than five."

"So we optimized all these functions in the body, and in less than a year, she opened up a restaurant with her son, who is a fabulous chef. It's now a five-star restaurant. Sally is just shy of 80 and she's still working in the restaurant. She's thinking of opening a second one, because that one's been so successful."

CASE STUDY TWO:
CARL HIT THE GAS INSTEAD OF THE BRAKE

"I was 56 when I started to get dementia," health writer Carl Lowe told me. "It was scary. I'd hit the gas instead of the brake. Just as I was about to crash into the car in front of me, I'd suddenly realize what I was doing."

"I couldn't even remember where I kept the silverware in my own kitchen. I knew I had to do something. Fortunately, my wife saw a study showing people with celiac disease can get cognitive problems from gluten."

"I cut out bread, cookies, anything with wheat, barley, rye. I gave up oatmeal and cakes. Within a week, I knew that was the problem. And I lost five pounds in three days."

"Looking back, I realize I had a brain issue my whole life. I had trouble doing advanced work in school, and it affected my emotional intelligence. I believe that celiac disease contributed to my heart problems, too."

"Now I'm on the paleo diet – no grains, no dairy, no soy. It's working for me. I eat fruit, veggies, organic meat, wild-caught fish, eggs, coconut oil, and extra virgin organic olive oil. I have a little dark chocolate every day. And I try to jog with my shirt off to get more vitamin D."

"My whole life has turned around. I've got the concentration to sit down and finish writing a novel. I can play guitar again. The arthritis has gone from all ten fingers to just one finger. I had dementia – and I recovered."

CASE STUDY THREE:
ROB STOPPED FUNCTIONING AFTER THREE CONCUSSIONS

When I looked at Rob, a fit, handsome business executive, I found it hard to believe this smiling man had suffered so much. But after multiple concussions playing sports, his brain was a mess. He was overly sensitive to noise and light. He couldn't sleep and he had trouble processing visual information, which made it hard to read. And his brain just felt tired.

For years, he wandered from doctor to doctor, seeking solutions in vain. Finally, he had the good fortune to discover Dr. Shari Caplan, a functional medicine specialist who founded the VitalityMD Clinic in Toronto, Canada.

"She said, 'Let's get your blood work done and see where the inefficiencies are. Then we can go through a supplement program. We can talk about diet and reducing inflammation.' It turned out I had a very high marker for inflammation. I had gone to a head injury clinic for four years, and they had never once talked to me about taking fish oil, reducing sugars and processed foods or taking supplements. The word 'inflammation' had never even come up!"

"My diet changed completely. I cut out gluten and put lots of avocados in my diet and coconut oil and curcumin and turmeric. I tried to sleep better and do light exercise. I worked at reducing stress with meditation, which I think is at the top of the list of tools to help recovery."

"I had hope again. And gradually over time, these changes got me back and gave me some focus. I still have challenges, but things have gotten quite a bit better. I'm still on this journey, trying to recover."

CASE STUDY FOUR:
KRISTIN WAS PATIENT ZERO

Kristin was in her early 60's when she noticed that she was starting to act like her late mother, who had suffered from Alzheimer's for 18 years. She got lost on the freeway, and could no longer analyze data at her job. As her situation deteriorated, she forgot her pets' names and the location of the light switches in her home.

"She'd been told by her physician that she had the same thing that her mother did. In fact, he wrote in the chart, "Memory problems," and so she was unable to get long term care insurance," Dr. Dale Bredesen, the author of *The End of Alzheimer's*, told me. "She actually called a friend and said that she was going to commit suicide, and her friend sent her here."

Kristin was Patient Zero, the first person that Dr. Bredesen treated with his ReCODE Protocol for Alzheimer's. Today, Dr. Bredesen is widely known as the doctor who made history with the first documented cases of reversing Alzheimer's disease. Kristin was his first success.

Dr. Bredesen's protocol includes a low-carb/healthy fats diet, exercise, sleep, supplements to cool down inflammation, treatment of toxic exposure and infections, balancing hormones, and online brain training. Since Kristin, he has used his protocol to treat hundreds of patients, and is now working to train 1,000 practitioners in his methods.

As for Kristin, she's now 73 and celebrating her fifth year of being on ReCODE. "She's doing absolute great, back at work full time. We're seeing this sort of thing again and again," Dr. Bredesen said.

CASE STUDY FIVE:
DEBBIE COULDN'T SPEAK, SWALLOW OR SEE

"Before I tried to commit suicide, I had so much to be grateful for, and I didn't even realize it," Debbie Hampton told me, in a deeply personal conversation. "When I got a second chance, I knew I had to heal my brain."

Today, Debbie is a vibrant and accomplished woman who writes about brain health on her excellent website (bestbrainpossible). But in 2007, Debbie tried to kill herself by taking pills. After a one-week coma, she awoke in a hospital. The pills had inflicted severe brain damage, and Debbie struggled to speak, swallow, and see. But something in Debbie fiercely wanted to live, and she committed herself to finding a brain-healing routine.

"More than one doctor told me I was wasting my time," Debbie said. "But the more I researched, the better I got. At first, I couldn't speak. So I'd visualize my brain making the connections for me to talk. I couldn't move my mouth, but I visualized it going through the alphabet, moving like it should."

Using Visualizations and Affirmations to Recharge the Brain

"That's a proven technique called visualization, based on neuroplasticity, the ability of the brain to adapt and make new connections. While I did my visualizations, I'd think positive thoughts in the present tense about what I wanted – that's an affirmation. So I'd visualize my speech as a flowing stream, while thinking, 'My speech is fluid, it flows naturally.'

"It got to the point where I'd discover a problem and knew where to focus. Anyone can use this method. For instance, if your hand shakes, visualize it being steady. I had my healing time every day, when I'd sit in a wicker chair by the window and practice meditation, visualizations and affirmations. I also exercised every day and cleaned up my diet. I ate protein and good fat like coconut oil. I drank lots of water and took fish oil and B vitamins and many other supplements.

Dramatic Results from Online Brain Training

"And every day for an hour, I did online brain training. The results were dramatic. I used the **Posit** program (www.brainhq.com) and my processing speed and vision got so much better. Hyperbaric oxygen chamber therapy helped a lot, too, and so did neurofeedback."

"We have to make the cognitive effort to focus on the good. The way you feel today lays down neuro-pathways that make it easier to think positive thoughts tomorrow."

"I'm extremely happy now and grateful. I realize that good health comes from your whole approach to life: what you eat, what you think, how you sleep, how you move your body. It's all about your relationship with yourself. I just thought of that. Eureka!"

ADDENDUM

DRUGS THAT HARM YOUR MEMORY

Many **medications** can negatively impact your brain, affecting cognitive function. These include **statins**, which are intended to lower lipids (cholesterol), and **anti-cholinergic drugs**.

Anti-cholinergics are designed to inhibit activity of acetylcholine, an essential neurotransmitter for memory and cognitive function. **Antihistamines, acid blockers, and antidepressants all are anti-cholinergic**, including several common over-the-counter drugs.

In addition to memory loss and cognitive impairment, anti-cholinergic drugs may cause nervousness, confusion, disorientation, hallucinations, restlessness, irritability, dizziness, drowsiness, blurred vision and light sensitivity.

Here is a list of drugs (prescription and over-the-counter) that can harm your memory and impair cognition. I want to thank Dr. Leo Galland, a renowned functional medicine specialist in New York, for graciously providing me with a complete list of anti-cholinergic drugs.

Remember: Don't stop taking medications without consulting your doctor.

STATINS
- Atorvastatin (Lipitor)
- Fluvastatin (Lescol, Lescol XL)
- Lovastatin (Mevacor, Altoprev)
- Pravastatin (Pravachol)
- Rosuvastatin (Crestor)
- Simvastatin (Zocor)
- Pitavastatin (Livalo)

Drugs with Anti-Cholinergic Properties (Courtesy of Dr. Leo Galland)
Some of these are available without prescription and may be found alone or combined with other drugs, especially in over-the-counter cold and headache remedies. Don't just rely on the product's name. Check all ingredients. Bring this information to your doctor.

Anti-spasmotics: used to relieve intestinal cramps or bladder symptoms, these are also found in numerous over-the-counter and prescription combination products used for colds and coughs, with various brand names:

- Atropine

- Belladonna (Donnatal and others)

- Clidinium (Quarzan)

- Dicyclomine (Bentyl and others)

- Flavoxate (Urispas)

- Glycopyrrolate (Robinul)

- Hyoscyamine (Levsin, NuLev, Cystospas and many others)

- Oxybutynin (Ditropan and others)

- Solifenacin (VesiCARE)

- Propantheline (ProBanthine and others)

- Scopolamine (Transderm-Scop and others)

- Tolterodine (Detrol)

- Trospium (Regurin and others)

Antihistamines: These are used in numerous over-the-counter and prescription products alone or in combination with other drugs for relieving symptoms of allergies, colds, dizziness, or improving sleep:

- Azatadine (Optimine and others)

- Chlorpheniramine (Chlortimeton and others)

- Clemastine (Contac, Tavist and others)

- Cyproheptadine (Periactin)

- Desloratadine (Clarinex and others)

- Dimenhydrinate (Dramamine and others)

- (Benadryl and many others)

- Doxylamine (Unisom and others)

- Hydroxyzine (Atarax, Vistaryl)

- Loratadine (Claritin and others)

- Meclizine (Antivert and others)

- Pyrilamine

Note: Fexofenadine (Allegra) and cetirizine (Zyrtec) are antihistamines that do not have anti-cholinergic effects, but may cause sedation.

Antacids: These are histamine H2 antagonists, used to relieve heartburn and stomach pain:

- Cimetidine (Tagamet)
- Famotidine (Pepcid)
- Nizatadine (Axid)
- Ranitidine (Zantac)

Note: Although these drugs have relatively weak anti-cholinergic activity, their use is associated with Mild Cognitive Impairment in older adults.

Antidepressants:

- Amitriptyline (Elavil and others)
- Amoxapine (Asendin)
- Citalopram (Celexa)
- Clomipramine (Anafranil)
- Desipramine (Norpramin)
- Doxepin (Sinequan and others)
- Duloxetine (Cymbalta)
- Escitalopram (Lexapro)
- Fluoxetine (Prozac)
- Imipramine (Tofranil)
- Lithium
- Nortriptyline (Pamelor, Aventyl)
- Paroxetine (Paxil and others)
- Protriptyline (Vivactil)

Muscle relaxants:

- Carisoprodal (Soma and others)
- Chlorzoxazone (Parafon Forte and others)
- Cyclobenzaprine (Flexeryl and others)
- Methocarbamol (Robaxin and others)
- Orphenadrine (Norflex and others)

Anti-arrythmics: used to treat cardiac arrhythmias:

- Digoxin
- Disopyramide (Norpace and others)
- Procainamide
- Quinidine (Quinaglute and others)

Anti-emetics: used to suppress nausea or vomiting:

- Promethazine (Phenergan and others)
- Prochlorperazine (Compazine and others)
- Trimethobenzamide (Tigan)

Antipsychotics: used for severe psychiatric disorders:

- Chlorpromazine (Thorazine and others)
- Clozapine (Clopine and others)
- Mesoridazine (Serentil)
- Olanzapine (Zyprexa)
- Promazine
- Quetiapine (Seroquel)
- Thioridazine (Mellaril)

Anti-parkinsonian: used in the treatment of Parkinson's disease and related disorders:

- Amantadine (Symmetrel)
- Benztropine (Cogentin)
- Biperiden (Akineton)
- Procyclidine (Kemadrine)
- Trihexyphenidyl (Artane and others)

Miscellaneous:

These drugs were shown to have anti-cholinergic effects at high concentration. They may exert clinically significant anti-cholinergic side effects when used at high doses or in people with impaired kidney function or a heightened susceptibility to anti-cholinergic side effects:

- Amoxicillin (an antibiotic)
- Carbamazepine (Tegretol, a drug for controlling seizures or chronic pain)
- Celecoxib (Celebrex, an anti-inflammatory pain reliever)
- Cephalexin (Keflex, an antibiotic)
- Diazepam (Valium, a tranquilizer)
- Diphenoxylate (Lomotil, a drug for diarrhea)
- Fentanyl (Duragesic, a narcotic pain reliever)
- Furosemide (Lasix, a diuretic used for fluid retention)
- Hydrocodone (a narcotic pain reliever, found in Vicodin)
- Lansoprazole (Prevacid, a proton pump inhibitor, used to reduce stomach acid)
- Levofloxacin (Levaquin, an antibiotic)
- Metformin (Glucophage, a drug that reduces blood sugar, used by diabetics)
- Phenytoin (Dilantin, a drug for controlling seizures)
- Temazepam (Restoril, a sleeping pill)
- Topiramate (Topimax, a drug used for preventing migraine headaches)

Anti-cholinergic eye drops may affect the brain. They are used to dilate the pupils. These include:

- Cyclopentolate
- Homatropine
- Tropicamide

Anti-cholinergic Herbs: Numerous herbs and natural products have anti-cholinergic effects and may be more hazardous than medications. Here are those that have been studied the most:

- Amanita muscaria (fly agaric)
- Amanita pantherina (panther mushroom)
- Arctium lappa (burdock root)
- Atropa belladonna (deadly nightshade)

- Cestrum nocturnum (night blooming jessamine)
- Datura metel (yangjinhua, used in traditional Chinese remedies)
- Datura suaveolens (angel's trumpet)
- Datura stramonium (jimson weed)
- Hyoscyamus niger (black henbane)
- Lantana camara (red sage)
- Phyllanthus emblica (Indian gooseberry)
- Solanum carolinensis (wild tomato)
- Solanum dulcamara (bittersweet)
- Solanum pseudocapsicum (Jerusalem cherry)

Know What You Are Taking

You should know everything that you or people in your family are taking: drugs and supplements and their potential side effects and interactions. If cognitive impairment is a problem and you're taking one or more of the substances listed above, what you're taking may be a cause or contributor.

HOW TO FIND A DOCTOR
AND OTHER RELEVANT RESOURCES

Academy of Integrative Health and Medicine
https://www.aihm.org/

Alternatives for Healing
http://www.alternativesforhealing.com/local-search-holistic-practitioners/

American Holistic Health Association (AHHA)
https://ahha.org/

Complementary and Alternative (CAM) subset of National Institutes of Health PubMed
https://nccih.nih.gov/research/camonpubmed

Explore Integrative Medicine
https://exploreim.ucla.edu/references/professional-associations/

Institute of Functional Medicine
https://www.ifm.org/

Metabolic Medical Institute
http://www.a4mfellows.net/

MPI Cognition (Dr. Dale Bredesen's protocol for reversing Alzheimer's)
https://www.mpicognition.com/

National Center for Complementary and Integrative Health
https://nccih.nih.gov/health/integrative-health